The neurobiological basis of psychiatric disorder is a rapidly expanding field of study, primarily as the result of recent developments in the basic neurosciences. *Neurobiology and Psychiatry* serves as an important forum for the evaluation and dissemination of information on this fundamental aspect of biological psychiatry. The topics selected for review illustrate the application of a range of modern neurobiological techniques to all the major psychiatric disorders. This, the third in the series, is devoted to the role and advances in neuroimaging within psychiatry. Earlier volumes have reviewed neurochemical and pathological issues and microhistology and molecular neurobiology, respectively. This series of up-to-date topic-orientated reviews of current research acts as an important information resource for all clinical and laboratory workers in the field.

Cambridge Medical Reviews

Neurobiology and Psychiatry Volume 3

Neuroimaging

Cambridge Medical Reviews provides regular volumes of critically selected review material in a growing range of emerging and established disciplines within clinical medicine. They concentrate particularly on areas where advances in basic biomedical science have a substantial contribution to make to the understanding and treatment of disease. Rigorous standards of selection and editing ensure a reliable, topical and clinically relevant series of volumes, focused to meet the requirements of clinicians and research workers in each discipline.

Neurobiology and Psychiatry

Contents of Volume 1

Post-mortem neurochemistry of schizophrenia, M C ROYSTON and M D C SIMPSON; Neurotransmitter system abnormalities associated with the neuropathology of Alzheimer's disease, D DEWAR; Temporal lobe pathology and schizophrenia, J M GOLD and D R WEINBERGER; Molecular neuropathology of Alzheimer's disease M GOEDERT, M C POTIER and M G SPILLANTINI; Neurochemical studies of cortical and subcortical dementias, A J CROSS; Subcortical dementia – defining a clinical syndrome, S FLEMINGER; Molecular and cell biology of epilepsy, B S MELDRUM and A G CHAPMAN; New developments in neuroimaging in schizophrenia, L S PILOWSKY and R KERWIN

Contents of Volume 2

Molecular genetics and the major psychoses, M GILL and C WALSH; Alzheimer's disease and the β-amyloid precursor protein, J HARDY; The biochemistry of tau proteins in Alzheimer's disease, J-M GALLO; Cytoarchitectonic and developmental studies in schizophrenia, P FALKAI and B BOGERTS; Neuroendocrine developments in psychiatric research, J A BEARN and P W RAVEN; From antibody to gene in schizophrenia: a review of the technology and a progress report, W G HONER and J L KENNEDY; Neurotrophins and neurodegenerative disease, D DAWBARN, S J ALLEN and H MACGOWAN; The biology of mental handicap, A J HOLLAND; HIV infection and the brain: an examination of clinical and pathological effects, I P EVERALL and P L LANTOS; Magnetic resonance spectroscopy: applications in psychiatry, M S KESHAVAN and J W PETTEGREW

Cambridge Medical Reviews

Neurobiology and Psychiatry
Volume 3
Neuroimaging

EDITOR

ROBERT KERWIN
Institute of Psychiatry, University of London, London, UK

ADVISORY EDITORS

DAVID DAWBARN
Department of Medicine, Bristol Royal Infirmary, Bristol, UK

JAMES McCULLOCH
Wellcome Surgical Institute and Hugh Fraser Neuroscience Laboratories, University of Glasgow, Glasgow, UK

CAROL TAMMINGA
Inpatient Program, Maryland Psychiatric Research Center, Baltimore, Maryland, USA

CAMBRIDGE
UNIVERSITY PRESS

CAMBRIDGE UNIVERSITY PRESS
Cambridge, New York, Melbourne, Madrid, Cape Town,
Singapore, São Paulo, Delhi, Tokyo, Mexico City

Cambridge University Press
The Edinburgh Building, Cambridge CB2 8RU, UK

Published in the United States of America by Cambridge University Press, New York

www.cambridge.org
Information on this title: www.cambridge.org/9780521203500

First published 1995
First paperback edition 2011

A catalogue record for this publication is available from the British Library

ISBN 978-0-521-45365-3 Hardback
ISBN 978-0-521-20350-0 Paperback

Contents

Contributors

BUSATTO, G F, Section of Clinical Neuropharmacology, Department of Psychological Medicine, Institute of Psychiatry, De Crespigny Park, Denmark Hill, London SE5 8AF, UK

DAVID, A, Department of Psychological Medicine, King's College Hospital, Denmark Hill, London SE5 9RS, UK

HARRISON, P J, University Department of Psychiatry, Warneford Hospital, and Department of Neuropathology, Radcliffe Infirmary, Oxford, UK

HOWARD, R, Department of Psychiatry of Old Age, Institute of Psychiatry, De Crespigny Park, Denmark Hill, London SE5 8AF, UK

LIDDLE, P F, Department of Psychiatry, University of British Columbia, 2255 Wesbrook Mall, Vancouver, Canada V6T 2A1

LOATS, H, Loats Associates Inc, PO Box 528, Westminster, Maryland 21158, USA

LOATS, S E, Loats Associates Inc, PO Box 528, Westminster, Maryland 21158, USA

PILOWSKY, L S, Department of Psychiatry, Institute of Psychiatry, De Crespigny Park, Denmark Hill, London SE5 8AF, UK

RIPPEON, T L, Loats Associates Inc, PO Box 528, Westminster, Maryland 21158, USA

SEIBYL, J P, Departments of Diagnostic Radiology and Psychiatry, Yale University School of Medicine, TE-2, 333 Cedar Street, New Haven, CT 06520, USA

SHARMA, T, Institute of Psychiatry, De Crespigny Park, Denmark Hill, London SE5 8AF, UK

WOODRUFF, P W R, Department of Psychological Medicine, Institute of Psychiatry, De Crespigny Park, Denmark Hill, London SE5 8AF, UK

Editor's preface

This is the third volume in the *Neurobiology and Psychiatry* series. As before, we have attempted to draw together comprehensive reviews of up-to-date neuroscience research by younger writers who are still very much hands-on in the field. In contrast to the first two disease-based volumes 1 and 2, this volume is more methodologically based and is devoted to neuroimaging. In this volume I have tried to encompass a complete spectrum of reviews from structural imaging, through functional MRI to PET and SPET, and was particularly keen to include a section on in vitro imaging, a topic often overlooked in the discipline of neuroimaging. I was also eager to include analytical chapters that are applicable to some imaging modalities.

Once again, I am grateful to Cambridge University Press for their continued support of this project and to my Personal Assistant, Pat O'Hara, for coordinating the project.

Robert W Kerwin
Reader in Clinical Neuropharmacology
Institute of Psychiatry
20.1.95

Abbreviations

AC–PC anterior commissure–posterior commissure
AD Alzheimer's disease
APP amyloid precursor protein
ASPECT annular single-crystal brain imaging system
ATP activation task profile

BOLD blood oxygenation level dependent contrast imaging

CBF cerebral blood flow
CT computerized tomography

DAT dementia of the Alzheimer type
DWMH deep white matter hyperintensity

EPI echoplanar imaging
EPS extrapyramidal side effect
ERP event-related brain potential
ETD eye tracking dysfunction

FLASH fast low angle shot
FWHF full-width half-maximum

GE gradient echo

ICC immunocytochemistry
ISHH in situ hybridization histochemistry

MRI magnetic resonance imaging
MZ monozygotic

NIMH National Institute of Mental Health

PCR polymerase chain reaction
PD Parkinson's disease
PET positron emission tomography

RF radiofrequency
ROI region of interest

SE spin–echo
SPET single-photon emission tomography

TE echo time
TI inversion time
TR repetition time

VBR ventricular brain ratio

WCST Wisconsin Card Sorting Test
WH white matter

Structural magnetic resonance imaging in psychiatry: the functional psychoses

P W R WOODRUFF

Introduction

Magnetic resonance imaging (MRI) is a means of detecting a spatially localized signal which arises from the magnetic property of atomic nuclei. Although the technique for inducing magnetic resonance was developed in 1946, it is only since the work of Lauterbur over 20 years later that magnetic resonance has been used to produce images[1]. Within a few years the clinical and research applications of this high resolution imaging technique were recognized. The technology is ever advancing to enable higher resolution images at faster acquisition time. MRI is now established as the gold standard in vivo technique for delineation of brain anatomy.

Principles of MRI

Magnetic properties of atomic nuclei

Mass, electrical charge and magnetism are basic properties of matter. Most mass is contained within the atomic nucleus. Each nucleus consists of protons (positively charged) and neutrons (no charge). Hydrogen is unique in having only one proton. The total number of protons and neutrons defines an isotope. Rotation of nuclei induces a magnetic field so that each nucleus becomes a dipole with north and south poles. The combined effect of the spin from multiple nuclei leads to the total spin property for each isotope. The application of an external magnetic field to an object interacts with the object's inherent nuclear spin to produce 'precession'. Precession is a cone-shaped rotating motion likened to that of a spinning gyroscope (Fig. 1). The frequency of precession is unique for each isotope, and increases in proportion to the magnetic field strength applied to it.

All correspondence to: Dr PWR Woodruff, Psychological Medicine, Institute of Psychiatry, De Crespigny Park, Denmark Hill, London SE5 8AF, UK.

Cambridge Medical Reviews: Neurobiology and Psychiatry Volume 3

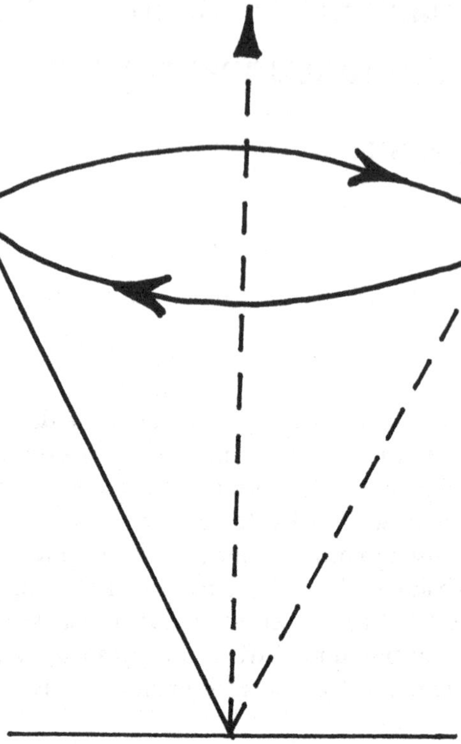

Fig. 1. Precession of an object around the vertical axis.

The MRI signal

The abundance of hydrogen in tissues makes its contribution to the MR signal particularly important. The hydrogen proton dipole is orientated either parallel or anti-parallel to the external magnetic field. Most protons adopt the low energy parallel position. When a radiofrequency impulse is applied, more protons move to the high energy anti-parallel position, a phenomenon known as resonance. Protons later resume the 'baseline' parallel position with the resultant release of radiofrequency energy. This energy is detected as the MR signal.

The combined magnetic effect of millions of atomic nuclei results in the measurable net magnetism of an object. The direction of net magnetism is described according to its orientation with respect to the externally applied magnetic field. The *xy* (transverse) plane is at right angles to the field and the *z* (longitudinal) plane is parallel to the external magnetic field. The *xy* plane can be considered to rotate around the *z* axis at the precessional frequency of the protons. This gives a stationary vector that describes the magnitude and direction of net magnetization in the transverse plane.

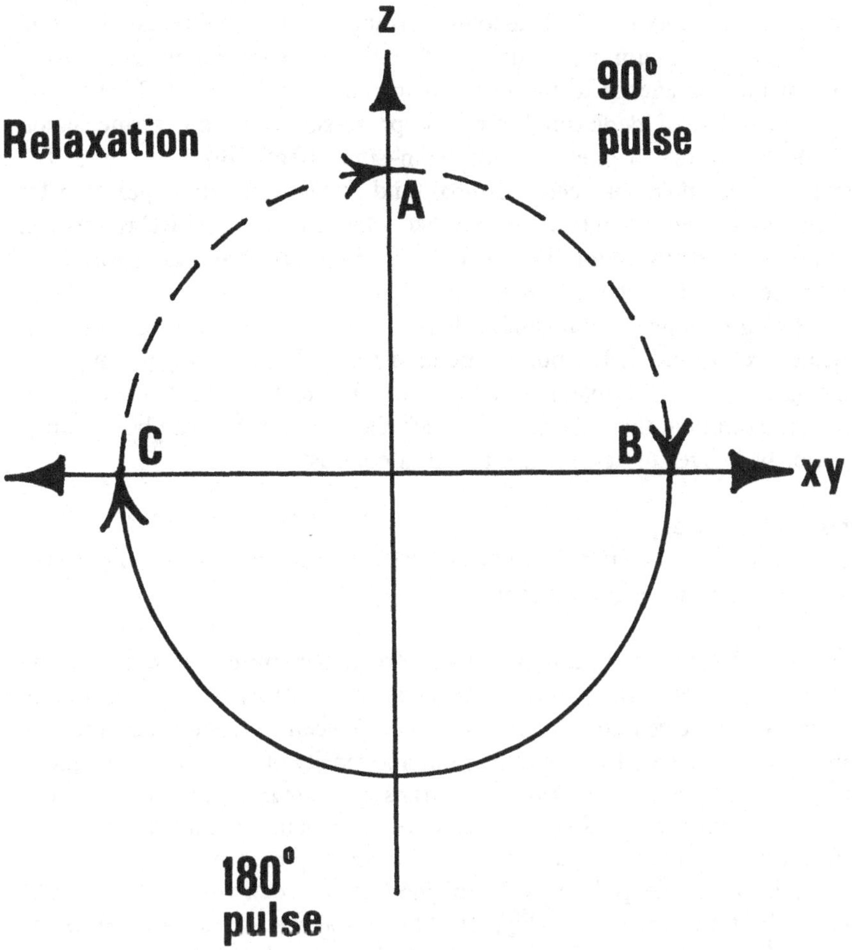

Fig. 2. Application of a radiofrequency pulse at the proton resonant frequency moves the net magnetization vector in the *xy* direction (A to B). A 180° spin–echo pulse refocuses the vector in the *xy* plane (C). Relaxation results in the magnetization vector then returning to the original position (A).

At rest, in an external magnetic field, net magnetization lies in the longitudinal *z* direction with none in the transverse *xy* plane. Application of a radiofrequency pulse (RF) at the proton resonant frequency in the transverse direction changes the net magnetization from the *z* to the *xy* direction (Fig. 2). A spin–echo pulse allows refocusing of the spins (see below). After the RF pulse stops, the magnetization vector returns to its original *z* direction by the process of relaxation. For a given tissue, relaxation in the longitudinal and transverse planes occurs at different rates described by the time constants T-1 and T-2. T-1 denotes relaxation in the longitudinal direction and T-2, relaxation in the transverse direction. T-1 relaxation results from loss of nuclear energy to the local environment or lattice. T-2 relaxation occurs because of 'dephasing' of proton precession causing net cancellation of the transverse magnetic vector (spin–spin effect). Both T-1 and T-2 relaxation for fluids like cerebrospinal fluid (csf) are much longer than for other tissues with higher fat content like white matter. The RF pulses can be altered so as to weight T-1 or T-2 relaxation times in such a way as to optimize contrast between the tissues of interest.

Imaging parameters that can be altered to maximize the contrast required include echo time (TE), pulse repetition time (TR), inversion time (TI) and flip angle of the magnetization vector. Different pulse sequences will be discussed first, then, the way in which these parameters can be modified to weight images to achieve the required contrast.

Imaging sequences

The most commonly used sequences for structural imaging are those called spin–echo and inversion recovery.

Spin–echo After the application of a radiofrequency impulse (RF pulse), the transverse signal decays due to dephasing of protons precessing in the *xy* plane. This decay is due to interference between neighbouring spinning protons (spin–spin effect) as well as inhomogeneity of the external magnetic field. The observed time of decay in transverse magnetization due to both of these effects is called T-2*. The spin–echo sequence maximizes the signal (otherwise lost due to dephasing) by 'refocusing' spins that are out of phase. An initial 90-degree pulse tips the magnetization vector from the longitudinal to the transverse plane (Fig. 3). This is followed by a 180-degree refocusing pulse which produces a recordable spin–echo at the time interval equal to that between the 90-degree and 180-degree pulses.

Inversion recovery spin–echo An initial 180-degree pulse inverts the magnetization vector in the *z* plane followed by the conventional spin–echo sequence of a 90-degree and 180-degree pulse sequence. The inversion time (TI) is the interval between the initial 180-degree pulse and the 90-degree pulse that follows. The signal largely depends on the extent of T-1 relaxation that has occurred during the inversion time and is therefore highly T-1 weighted. The disadvantage of inversion recovery is long imaging time and hence the potential for movement artefact. Reducing imaging time by lessening the number of data acquisitions is at the expense of the signal-to-noise ratio. Physiological movement can be taken into account by cardiac or respiratory gating. Faster imaging techniques, e.g. gradient echo pulse sequences, have particular uses in blood flow angiography and for detecting csf pulsation.

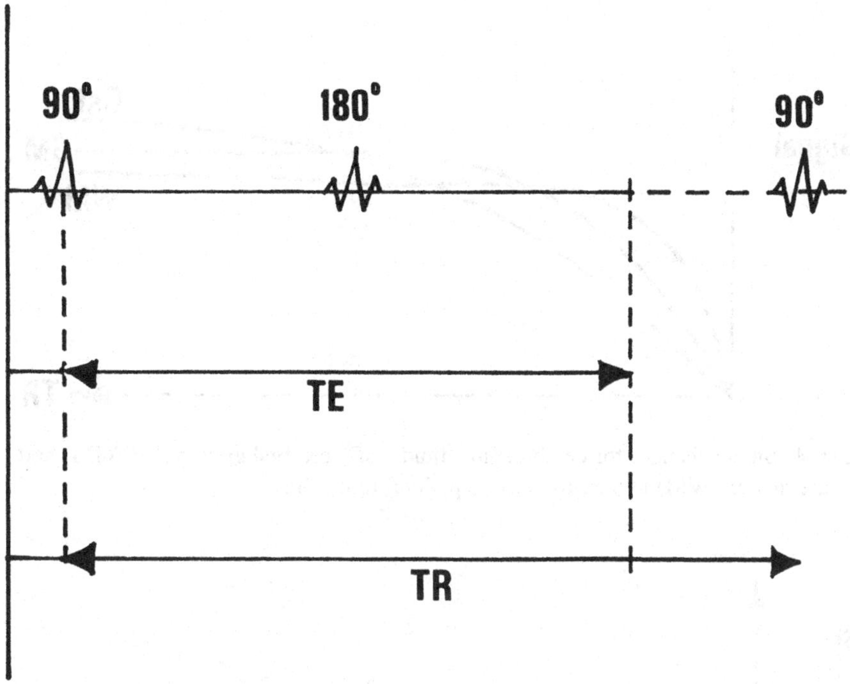

Fig. 3. The pulse sequence of the spin–echo. TE = echo time; TR = pulse repetition time.

Ultra-fast techniques like echo planar imaging are increasingly being applied for functional imaging.

T-1 and T-2 contrast The T-1 and T-2 values for csf, white and grey matter are shown in Table 1. Signal changes due to variations in TR are dependent on T-1 relaxation rates. As seen in Fig. 4, tissues with short T-1, e.g. white matter (WM), give a bright signal at short TR intervals. At long TR, the signal depends increasingly on proton density, and so the csf signal becomes more prominent. Signal intensity also varies with TE. The interrelationship between the effects of TR on the signal are shown in Fig. 5.

Table 1. *T-1 and T-2 relaxation times for the three main brain tissues are shown in seconds*

Tissue	T-1	T-2
Cerebrospinal fluid	4.0	2.0
Grey matter	1.0	0.08
White matter	0.6	0.03

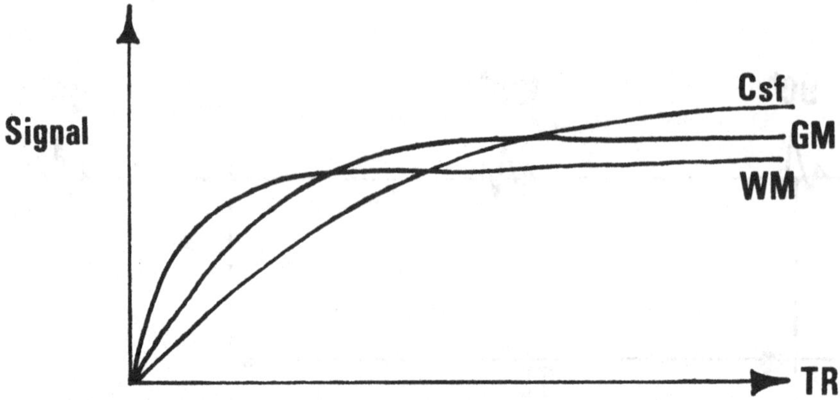

Fig. 4. Signal changes for cerebrospinal fluid (csf), cerebral grey matter (GM) and white matter (WM) at varying pulse repetition times (TR).

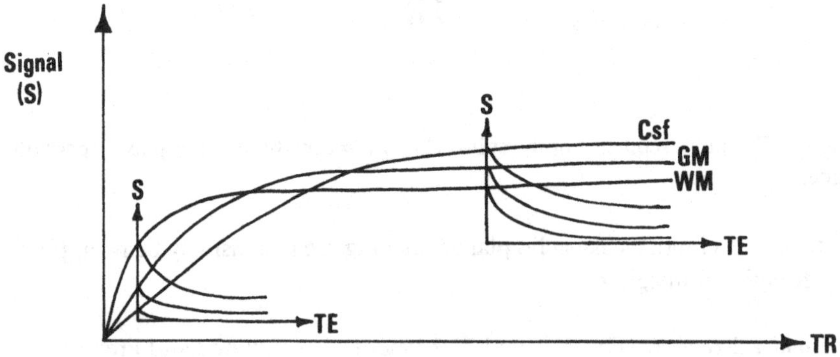

Fig. 5. Signal changes for cerebrospinal fluid (csf), cerebral grey matter (GM) and white matter (WM) at varying pulse repetition times (TR), both at short and long echo times (TE).

At short TR and TE, signal contrast is T-1 weighted, being greater from tissues with short T-1 characteristics. At long TR and TE the signal is T-2 weighted, so tissues with longer T-2 characteristics give a brighter signal. At long TR and short TE the signal depends on proton density, hence the prominent signal from csf.

Thus in T-1 weighted images, tissues with short T-1 values give high signal density (white matter > grey matter > csf). In T-2 weighted images, tissues with long T-2 values give high signal intensity (csf > grey matter > white matter). In proton density images, tissues with high water content give a large signal.

Volumetric analysis

Many studies using MRI in psychiatry measure volume or areas of anatomical regions. High resolution plus appropriate imaging sequences are required to maximize contrast. In general, resolution has improved considerably in recent years with the use of more powerful magnets and more refined hardware. Early studies using planimetry and simple linear or area measures have evolved to more accurate volume measurements with computer-outlining techniques. Usually slices of 1–10 mm thick are taken, and the anatomical region is outlined and volume estimated from the area multiplied by slice thickness. The thinner the slice, the better the estimate of volume as long as resolution is adequate. However, as the slice becomes thinner, the signal/noise ratio is reduced. There is, therefore, the need to balance these factors which depend on the technology available.

The importance of MRI in psychiatry

Clinical applications

Clinical applications of MRI include: 1) diagnosis of organic brain disorders; 2) monitoring progress of chronic disorders; and 3) assessing prognosis. MRI is more sensitive than computerized tomography (CT) at detecting non-calcified intracranial lesions and gives much better anatomical detail. MRI complements CT in aiding diagnosis of physical brain disease that underlies organic psychoses, e.g. cerebral infarction or tumour. Clinical indications for MRI in psychiatric patients are similar to those for CT and include: 1) history of head injury or other neurological disease; 2) presence of neurological signs including movement disorder of unknown cause; 3) acute confusion or gradual cognitive decline; 4) dementia; and 5) first psychosis or major personality change in patients over 50 years old[2].

MRI is the most sensitive technique for detecting small lesions such as hyperintensities or microinfarcts as may be seen in temporal arteritis or systemic lupus erythematosis. White matter lesions on T-2 weighted images may be important in the clinical assessment of multiple sclerosis. Plaque count relates to prognosis in this condition. Diffuse white matter changes such as leucoencephalopathy in AIDS can be seen clearly using MRI. Because of its sensitivity, MRI may demonstrate cerebral atrophy before obvious cognitive decline in patients with dementing illnesses including AIDS. Specific regions may be more easily identified with MRI than CT, like the pituitary gland in neuroendocrinological conditions. It may be preferable to use MRI on patients with conditions like AIDS when multiple pathology is suspected like atrophy, leucoencephalopathy and intracranial lesions like lymphoma or toxoplasmosis.

MRI does not expose patients to X-ray radiation, and, as long as there are no contra-indications, is safer than CT. Contra-indications to MRI include: 1) metallic implants, e.g. aneurysm clips or orthopaedic screws; 2) metallic foreign bodies, e.g. metal lathe eye injuries or shotgun injuries; and 3) pregnancy.

Research applications

The importance of MRI in psychiatric research is to enable expansion of post-mortem and CT brain studies by providing the means to measure neuroanatomical regions in vivo. Furthermore, MRI can detect boundaries between grey and white matter within anatomical regions. Combining structural MRI with information using clinical, neuropsychological, neurophysiological and functional neuroimaging techniques provides a powerful means of detecting important relationships between brain structure and function in psychiatry.

Subject selection in MRI studies

Much has been learnt about normal brain morphology from MRI studies in psychiatry that use a normal control group for comparison. Brain abnormality can be defined by significant deviation from a normal control range. Therefore, it is important to: 1) determine normal brain morphology; and 2) identify features of subject groups that may influence the brain structures being studied. For instance, schizophrenia may be a heterogeneous condition in which only subgroups of patients have brain abnormalities. The finding of statistically significant differences in size of brain structures between schizophrenics and controls may therefore depend on the criteria used to select the two groups. The choice of control subjects is therefore crucial to MRI studies which draw conclusions often from small differences between groups.

The normal brain

Normal brain asymmetry

The left occipital pole is larger and extends more posteriorly than the right, whereas the right frontal region is often larger and protrudes more anteriorly than does the left. The right temporal region is usually larger than the left. Compared with the right, on the left side, the planum temporale is larger and the Sylvian fissure ascends more steeply and extends more posteriorly[3].

In general, men show more hemispheric asymmetry than women[4]. The corpus callosum is possibly larger and more bulbous posteriorly in women and non-right-handers[5,6]. Right-handed persons may have more cerebral asymmetry than left-handers[7]. Cerebral size in women is less than men. This difference is probably related to factors determining height[8].

Age
Brain shrinkage, in the absence of cognitive deficit, is more noticeable as age advances. This shrinkage becomes more prominent after the age of 55. Studies using MRI have demonstrated age-related decreases in volume of cerebral cortex, cortical grey matter, basal ganglia and anterior diencephalic grey matter[9,10]. Murphy[11] compared two groups of subjects aged < 35 and > 60 and found specific reduction in lenticular and caudate nuclei, after taking reduced cerebral size into account. Volume of lateral ventricles, third ventricle and csf were all greater in the older group. Normal brain asymmetry was preserved. Similar results have been described in other studies[12].

Social class
A negative association has been found between socioeconomic status and brain size[13]. It has been suggested that this association may be due to poor nutrition adversely affecting brain growth. The association may also be due to the fact that people with conditions that result in brain shrinkage 'drift' down the social scale as a result of their condition. Using paternal social class to match subject groups may take account of social drift.

Intelligence and education
Intelligence accounts for about 12–30% of the variance in brain size of normal individuals, being greater the higher the IQ. Andreasen[14] found IQ correlated with volumes of cerebrum, cerebellum, temporal lobe, hippocampus and grey matter. There was no such correlation with white matter, cerebrospinal fluid, caudate or lateral ventricular volume. The finding of decreased frontal lobe size in schizophrenics was later attributed to the choice of a control group with more years of education[8]. Comparison of the same patient group with a control group matched for education did not reveal differences in frontal lobe size[15].

The abnormal brain

Factors affecting brain structure

Injury MRI is very sensitive to lesions which may persist after full clinical recovery from trauma. There may, for example, be distinct foci or more generalized atrophy observed. Special care needs to be exercised in evaluating individuals likely to have such lesions before including them in research study groups.

Pre-existing neuropsychiatric disease Many neuropsychiatric diseases are associated with significant brain abnormalities detectable using MRI. Common examples include: Parkinson's disease, Alzheimer's disease, multi-infarct dementia, AIDS, systemic lupus erythematosis and multiple sclerosis.

Alcohol Psychiatric disorder amongst alcoholics and drug abusers is common. One study of alcoholics demonstrated that 65% had a current psychiatric disorder including antisocial personality disorder (36.5%), affective disorder (27%), schizophrenia (4.3%)[16]. It is, therefore, particularly likely that studies on psychiatric patients will include alcoholics and drug abusers[17]. From an emergency clinic sample, 47% of schizophrenics had a lifetime risk of alcohol abuse-related disorder[18].

Post-mortem studies have demonstrated loss of cerebral and cerebellar cortical neurones and white matter in alcoholics. Female alcoholics are more likely to develop these changes[19,20]. However, it was demonstrated in a recent post-mortem study that, although compared with controls, alcoholic male brains were smaller, they contained the same number of neurones[21]. MRI studies in alcoholics demonstrate reversible and irreversible brain shrinkage. Zipursky et al[22] demonstrated reversibility of ventricular enlargement after abstinence.

Raised T-1 level was related to cognitive impairment in some alcoholics[23]. More detailed studies in alcoholics have demonstrated volume reductions in cortical and subcortical cerebral structures. These structures include: diencephalon, caudate nucleus, dorsolateral prefrontal and parietal cortices and medial temporal lobe regions. Cortical and ventricular csf was increased. Cerebral grey matter was reduced[24]. Generalized grey and white matter loss was more marked in older than younger alcoholics with equivalent drinking history. This was interpreted as an age-related increase in vulnerability of the brain to effects of chronic alcohol abuse[25].

Other substances Opiates, cocaine, solvents, benzodiazephines and other drugs or chemicals may also be related to brain abnormalities[26–28]. It is, therefore, prudent to take account of drug abuse in studies designed to investigate brain abnormalities from other causes.

Previous treatment There is little evidence that neuroleptic medication per se alters brain structure detectable using MRI except perhaps the basal ganglia. Studies in psychotic patients do not generally find correlations between brain size and length of exposure to, or dose of, anti-psychotics[29].

Structural brain abnormalities in patients referred for ECT include lateral and third ventricular enlargement, atrophy of frontal and temporal lobes, amygdala and hippocampus. On the evidence available it seems unlikely that ECT itself results in progression of these abnormalities[30]. T-1 values may rise acutely after ECT and return to normal within hours. The rise in T-1 level probably represents temporary disruption of the blood–brain barrier[31].

Schizophrenia

Ventricular size

One of the most consistent findings using structural brain imaging of schizophrenic patients has been that of increased lateral ventricular size (Table 2). Increased third and fourth ventricular size has also been demonstrated in schizophrenia. Ventricular size has been traditionally expressed as the ventricular brain ratio (VBR) derived from the area of ventricles seen on a slice divided by the brain area on the same slice. The problem with this method is: 1) that VBR is altered by brain shrinkage; and 2) it assumes a linear relationship between ventricle and brain size. Also, ventricular size varies regionally such that left occipital and right posterotemporal horns are largest[32]. So, studies that only take measurements from a few slices can give misleading results. For these reasons it is better to measure whole ventricular size and statistically co-vary for the effects of whole brain volume[33]. Using such a technique, Kelsoe[34] found a 62% greater lateral ventricular volume and 73% larger third ventriclar volume in schizophrenics compared with normal controls. Degreef[32] measured the entire ventricular system in 40 patients with their first episode of schizophrenia. Lateral ventricular volume was 26% greater than normal controls, particularly in the left temporal and frontal horns. Left temporal horn volumes correlated with positive and negative symptoms including hallucinations, bizarre behaviour, affective flattening, attention deficit and anhedonia. Other studies have found correlations between lateral and third ventricular enlargement and positive symptoms[35]. Lateral ventricular volume in schizophrenics also correlate with negative symptoms[15]. Andreasen et al[15] did not demonstrate an association between ventricular size and age of onset of schizophrenia, duration and number of hospital admissions, cognitive impairment or previous neuroleptic treatment. Increased ventricular size has been related to poor outcome[36].

Generally, ventricular enlargement is more pronounced in male rather than female schizophrenics. The range of ventricular size is also usually greater in schizophrenic than in control groups[15,36]. Males tend to have larger ventricles than females in patient and control groups, thus confirming the sexual dimorphic characteristics of this in common with other brain regions[32].

The ventricular region is surrounded by areas such as the amygdala, hippocampus and parahippocampal gyrus. These structures contain neuronal networks concerned with selection, association and integration of sensory information, memory and control of basic drives and emotions. Reduced size of these areas has been demonstrated in schizophrenia and it is generally

Table 2. *MRI studies of brain regions in schizophrenics versus normal controls*

Study	Number of patients	Number of controls	M/F patients	Brain vol/area	VBR/ vent size	Left temp lobe	Right temp lobe	Corpus callosum	Front lobe	Hippo/ amygdala
1	18	18	11/7	<				>		
2	38	41	28/10					>		
3	38	49	28/10	>m					>*	
4	29	21	5/24		>					
5	20	20	15/5	>*	4=			<*		
6	27	14	22/5	<	L>*	<	<	<	R>, L=	>
7	15	15	15/0	>	>*			<		
8	35	25	22/13			>	>			L<m*
9[2]	24	25	11/9	>				<		
10[2]	21	21	15/6	>	>	<, L<R*	<			
11	12	12	8/4	<	>* 4>			<*		
12	15	15	15/0	<	3>	STG<*	STG<*			<, <L*
13	12	12	5/7	<				>		
14	28	21	15/13	<m	>, 3m>	<	<			R, L<m L<f
15	56	35	41/15	<	<m, <f 3>				<	
16[8]	15	18	9/6	<f				<m		
17	17	13	10/7	>	>	<*	<*	=	<	
18	15	15	8/7		>, 3>	WM< GM<*	WM> GM<		WM< GM<	R<* L<*

19[1]	15	20	9/6	<	>, 3>	<	<			<
20	42	43	27/15	<m, <f	>m, >f					
21	42	24	28/14	<	>					
22	31	33	24/7	<	>, 3>	<	>	<	>	=
23	44	29	19/15	<					WM<*	<*
24	72	31	49/23		L>* 3>					
25	40	25	25/15		L>R, 3>					
26	25	17	13/12	>		<*				
27	15	15	15/0	GM>, WM>	>, 3< 4<	<STG*	NS			<*
28	22	20	22/0	GM<* WM>	>*, 3>	GM<*	GM<*		GM<*	
29	48	34	37/11	<	L>* f>m R>f R<m	GM< WM<	GM< WM<			
30	30	44	23/7	<m*				<*m		

[1]Matthew (1985); [2]Nasrallah (1985); [3]Andreasen (1986); [4]Smith (1987); [5]Stratta (1987); [6]Kelsoe (1988); [7]Rossi (1988); [8]Bogerts (1989); [9]Hauser (1989); [10]Johnstone (1989); [11]Rossi (1989); [12]Barta (1990); [13]Casanova (1990); [14]Dauphinais (1990); [15]Nasrallah (1990); [16]Raine (1990); [17]Rossi (1990); [18]Suddath (1990); [19]DeLisi (1991); [20]Gur (1991); [21]Jernigan (1991); [22]Young (1991); [23]Breier (1992); [24]Bornstein (1992); [25]Degreef (1992); [26]di Michele (1992); [27]Sheraton (1992); [28]Zipursky (1992); [29]Harvey (1993); [30]Woodruff (1993).

[1]Neurological controls; [2]studies that included an affective disorder patient group.

L = left, R = right, m = males, f = females, GH = grey matter, WM = white matter, STG = superior temporal gyrus, * = statistically significant.

assumed that increased ventricular size reflects reduced size of surrounding brain regions. If so, ventricular size should correlate inversely with surrounding regions. This has not been the case in most studies[34].

That ventricular enlargement is often found in patients shortly after their first psychotic illness suggests that these brain abnormalities are longstanding. The lack of correlation between ventricular size and duration of illness further suggests non-progression of structural brain abnormalities once symptoms develop[35]. As foetal brain tissue expands, the proportion of ventricle to brain volume decreases. Therefore, increased VBR in schizophrenia *may* represent incomplete brain maturation or atrophy of surrounding regions.

Whole brain

Reduced cerebral size has been demonstrated in most MRI studies of schizophrenia (Table 2). Alterations in whole brain size are not necessarily equal to those of constituent regions. For example, Barta[37] found a 2% decrease in whole brain as opposed to that of 7–10% in temporal lobes. Mid-brain and pontine areas were actually increased in schizophrenics by 8% and 11%, respectively. Whole brain volumes were greater in schizophrenics than in controls despite reductions in superior temporal gyrus volume[38]. There may be an inverse relationship between csf fluid and brain volume in schizophrenics. Harvey[39] found overall decreases in cerebral volume and a corresponding increase in sulcal fluid volume in schizophrenics. A selective decrease in cortical volume accounted for the smaller cerebral volume.

Reductions in brain volume more often affect male than female schizophrenics[39]. Males accounted for the significance of reduced mid-sagittal brain areas in schizophrenics compared with normal controls[40]. The normal relationship between height and brain size may be lost in male schizophrenics. Cerebral size is less despite preservation of height[13].

Frontal lobe

There are reasons why investigating frontal lobe function is important in schizophrenia: 1) there may be clinical similarities between patients with frontal lobe damage and schizophrenic patients, particularly those with negative symptoms. For example, patients with frontal lobe lesions have deficits of attention, abstract thinking, judgement, motivation, affect and emotion, impulse control, as well as decreased spontaneous speech, verbal fluency and voluntary motor behaviour. 2) Schizophrenics may show impaired performance on neuropsychological tasks that require adequate frontal lobe function[41]. 3) Evidence supports frontal lobe underactivity during activation tasks in schizophrenia[42]. There may, therefore, be links between frontal lobe underactivity and underlying brain structure.

Most studies that have looked at frontal lobe size in schizophrenics demonstrate a reduction, although only a minority demonstrate that this is statistically significant. The first of these looked at mid-sagittal areas[8]. Failure to replicate these findings in comparison with a control group matched by educational level was interpreted as a negation of the previous finding[15]. Evidence that frontal lobe volume is reduced in schizophrenic groups is inconsistent[15,29,34,43]. Studies looking at neuropsychological deficits associated with frontal lobe activity have found relationships with frontal lobe size. For instance, common-sense judgement correlated with reduced frontal lobe volume in schizophrenics[44]. It may be, therefore, that only those patients with frontal lobe abnormalities have functional deficits in tasks that rely on frontal lobe function. Furthermore, frontal lobe deficits may arise from abnormalities in other brain regions connected to the frontal lobe. For example, underactivity of dorsolateral prefrontal cortex in schizophrenia during tasks requiring working memory was related to hippocampal volume[42]. Neural networks connecting these two regions may be functionally defective in schizophrenia. A deficiency of such neuronal connections may explain the observation that frontal lobe volume reduction was mainly confined to white matter[43]. Increased T-2 levels in white matter of the left frontal region also indicate white matter abnormalities in the frontal region[45].

Temporal lobes, hippocampus and amygdala

The finding of enlarged temporal horns of the lateral ventricles in schizophrenia has led researchers to measure temporal lobe structures that surround this ventricular region. A twin study that found lateral and third ventricular enlargement in schizophrenic co-twins also found reduced volume of left temporal lobe grey matter and hippocampal volume[29]. That temporal lobe volume remains constant in schizophrenia is supported by a lack of correlations between its volume and both the amount of exposure to neuroleptic medication and duration of illness. This stability is further confirmed by studies of patients with first onset of psychosis who also have abnormal medial temporal lobe morphology[46]. Sex differences are confirmed by the finding of left-sided changes more frequently seen in male schizophrenics[47].

In young acute schizophrenics temporal lobe reduction may be lateralized to the left side[48]. Patients with familial schizophrenia who are genetically predisposed also have smaller temporal lobes. Reduction of 10% in temporal lobe size has been observed in such a group of patients[49]. However, there are studies that have not demonstrated significantly reduced temporal lobe volumes[34].

Of particular clinical relevance are findings suggestive of associations between psychiatric symptoms and brain structure. Some preliminary evidence supports specific left-sided temporal lobe abnormalities in regions relevant to auditory function. Barta et al[37] found decreased superior temporal gyrus volume to be associated selectively with auditory hallucinations. The superior temporal gyrus is an auditory association area, stimulation of which can result in complex auditory hallucinations. It has been argued that abnormalities of the superior temporal gyrus may be related to auditory hallucinations in schizophrenia. Shenton et al[38] described localized reductions of grey mater of the left temporal lobe in schizophrenics. Degree of thought disorder was related to volume reduction of the left posterior superior temporal gyrus. Rossi et al[50] noted reduced length of the planum temporale on the left in schizophrenics. This area is situated in the auditory association cortex.

Basal ganglia

Enlarged caudate nuclei have been described in a group of first onset schizophrenia-like patients[46]. Breier[43] found the left caudate nucleus enlarged in schizophrenics. Other studies do not confirm these findings[34]. Young[35] found reduced caudate size correlated with negative symptoms.

The lenticular nucleus and putamen may also be enlarged[51]. It is difficult to explain why some structures should be enlarged owing to a pathological process which may also result in reduced size of other brain regions. The replication and significance of these findings need clarification. Explanations for reduced size of basal ganglia structures, like abnormalities of synaptic pruning or compensatory increased synaptic density due to decreased input from other brain areas, remain speculative[46]. The effect of medication on basal ganglia structure also needs clarification.

The corpus callosum

A significant number of studies of schizophrenic subjects have measured the corpus callosum[40]. Its role in allowing integration of information from both cerebral hemispheres makes it a structure of theoretical importance in schizophrenia in which 'splitting' of psychic functions occurs. Evidence of abnormal inter-hemispheric communication in schizophrenia is provided by a number of neuropsychological studies. For instance, some schizophrenics show impaired ability in performing tasks that rely on transferring information from one hemisphere to the other[52,53].

Lewis first demonstrated an association between psychosis and dysgenesis of the corpus callosum[54]. Using MRI, Swayze et al[55] reported a significantly greater prevalence of corpus callosum agenesis in 140 schizophrenic patients than in controls. Another lesion related developmentally to the corpus callosum is cavum septum pellucidum. The association between this and schizophrenia was also first noted by Lewis[56]. In a further study, this lesion was detected in 21% of schizophrenics on MRI scans compared with 2% of controls[32]. These associations suggest that neurodevelopmental damage to the corpus callosum may predispose to the later onset of psychosis[54].

In view of evidence of callosal dysfunction in schizophrenia, and the association between developmental abnormalities of the corpus callosum and psychosis, morphological changes of the corpus callosum might be expected in schizophrenia. Deficient function due to neuronal loss, demyelination or failed development might be reflected in altered size. Stimulated by early post-mortem studies reporting increased corpus callosum size in schizophrenics and aided by the ease of its anatomical delineation, MRI studies focused on the corpus callosum[57]. Early studies used linear measures of width and length which mostly found no significant differences between schizophrenics and controls, although there was a suggestion that length was increased. The number of subjects in these studies may have been too small to pick up small differences. In addition, early studies did not account for differences of corpus callosum size and shape between males and females. It has been suggested that in the normal population, females have a larger splenium than males[5]. In schizophrenics, increased widths were found predominantly in females[58,59]. It has been shown that reduced corpus callosum area was confined to male schizophrenics[40]. Handedness also influences corpus callosum size. Witelson[6] found larger corpus callosum areas in right-handed individuals on post-mortem examination. Nasrallah[58] found MRI measurements of the corpus callosum area greater in right-handed, compared with left-handed, male schizophrenics.

Linear measures are particularly variable when applied to structures with differing outline like the corpus callosum. Therefore, area measures are probably more suitable. Most studies that have measured corpus callosum area show this to be less in schizophrenics compared with controls (Table 2). Taking account of brain size by calculating a ratio of corpus callosum to brain area is constrained by the same problems as apply to VBR[33]. The study using analysis of co-variance to account for effects of brain size found significantly reduced corpus callosum area in schizophrenics[35]. Area reduction was particularly reduced in that part of the corpus callosum that contains fibres connecting the two superior temporal gyri, the region whose volume reduction was associated with auditory hallucinations in schizophrenia[37]. In contrast, Gunther[60] found positive symptoms associated with larger, and negative symptoms with smaller, corpora callosa in schizophrenics.

Associations have also been found between reduced corpus callosum size and increased VBR[48]. Casanova[61] found a significantly altered shape of the corpus callosum in schizophrenics that related to ventricular size.

Overall, evidence favours reduced area of the corpus callosum in schizophrenia, predominantly in males. The clinical significance of these findings has still to be evaluated.

Major affective disorders

Studies using MRI have furthered knowledge already gained with CT and neuropathological techniques to investigate brain abnormalities in affective disorder. In particular, more specific quantitative evaluations of structural abnormalities and more sensitive detection of lesions has been possible with MRI. There are, however, difficulties in distinguishing image findings from the effects of ageing in patients. This difficulty is compounded by the association between cerebrovascular disease and affective disorder[62].

Volumes of brain structures

A number of MRI studies report ventricular enlargement and cortical atrophy, especially in elderly depressed patients. Temporal lobe size reduction, reported in at least one study of patients with affective disorder[63], was not confirmed in another[36]. Coffey et al[64] found reduced volume of cerebrum, frontal and temporal lobes, amygdala and hippocampus and increase in lateral and third ventricle volume in depressed patients. However, only frontal lobe volume was significantly decreased in depressed patients after adjustment for age, sex, education and cranial size. Coffman et al[65] found no difference in sagittal frontal lobe areas between young bipolar patients and controls.

It has been suggested that reduction in brain tissue in depressed patients could be due to hypercortisolaemia secondary to overactivity corticotrophin releasing factor from the pituitary. Pituitary enlargement as demonstrated by MRI in depressed patients is consistent with this hypothesis[62].

Reports of lateral and third ventricular enlargement in studies of patients with bipolar and unipolar illness have been inconsistent[64]. It may be that only those patients with cognitive impairment demonstrate ventricular enlargement, as has been demonstrated in association with cerebral atrophy[65].

Bilateral reduction of caudate volume has been demonstrated in a group of patients with major depression after considering the effects of age[66]. Degeneration of striatal neurones or terminals could lead to disrupted pathways involved in mood regulation.

Alteration of other brain structures in patients with affective disorder include reports of a smaller brain stem and cerebellar vermis[67].

MRI hyperintensities

T-2 weighted MR images reveal hyperintensities also known as unknown bright objects or 'UBOs'. These features correspond to hypodensities noted on CT scans. Hyperintensities have been detected in periventricular or deep white matter and subcortical grey matter. Hyperintensities are thought to result from a variety of degenerative brain changes including atherosclerosis, arteriolar hyalinization, lacunar infarcts, atrophic demyelination and leakage of csf into periventricular spaces. These supposed lesions are more prevalent in older depressed patients with risk of cardiovascular disease[68]. A number of studies have found increased frequency and size of hyperintensities in deep white matter (DWMHs) and subcortical nuclei in elderly patients with depression and in patients with bipolar disorder[64]. In a study of elderly depressed patients, 62% had periventricular hyperintensities compared with 23% in controls, 55% had deep white matter hyperintensities compared with 14% of controls and basal ganglia lesions were present in 51% of patients and only 5% of controls[69]. The occurrence of these lesions was associated with risk of cerebrovascular disease. To take account of cardiovascular risk factors, Figiel et al[70] compared early and late onset depressed patients with a control group well matched for cardiovascular risk factors. Basal ganglia lesions and large DWMHs were more commonly seen in late onset depressives than depressives of early onset.

Hyperintensity lesions are prevalent in those referred for ECT. Coffey et al[71] found 94% of referrals had periventricular hyperintensities, 77%, DWMHs, 34%, hyperintensities in the basal ganglia and thalamus and 23%, in the pons.

The clinical significance of hyperintensities is unknown. Hyperintensities may be related to cognitive impairment, poorer response to treatment and increased sensitivity to medication and ECT[62].

In contrast to unipolar disorder, young patients with bipolar disorder often have DWMHs. For instance, Figiel[70] demonstrated DWMHs in 44% bipolars compared with 6% of controls. These lesions were mainly located in the frontal and parietal lobe deep white matter.

Conclusions and future directions

MRI studies have contributed a great deal to the evidence that structural brain abnormalities underlie the functional psychoses. This evidence is particularly strong in schizophrenia. Patterns of structural brain abnormalities that have emerged include: 1) generalized diminution in cerebral size; 2) regional abnormalities of the temporal lobes and hippocampi; and 3) asymmetrical patterns such as left-sided temporal lobe abnormalities. Alteration of brain morphology is more apparent in male than female schizophrenics. The high resolution of MRI has enabled the detection of grey and white matter differences within cerebral regions. Also, hyperintensities are commonly detected in patients with major affective disorders. As MRI enables us to look at the brain in closer detail, so our understanding of factors that influence brain structure has increased, e.g. age and sex. Also, as a result of MRI work, the normal variation in brain size and shape has become more apparent. This knowledge allows us to improve study designs by taking account of factors that affect brain morphology. Advanced technology like computerized '3D rendering' and 'cerebral parcelation' will allow individual differences of cerebral anatomy to be accounted for more accurately in the future.

An important area of current and future research lies in linking structural and functional brain abnormalities. Already some links have been made between cerebral anatomy detected by MRI and clinical symptoms, e.g. size of the superior temporal gyrus and auditory hallucinations in schizophrenia. Sciences concerned with brain function are increasingly being used in conjunction with structural MRI of the brain. These disciplines include neuropsychology, neurophysiology and functional neuroimaging. The newest technique of functional neuroimaging, functional MRI, now provides the first opportunity to perform structural and functional measures in the same subject at the same sitting. The study of the relationship between brain structure and function is entering a new chapter.

Acknowledgements

I gratefully acknowledge the help of Dr Christine Heron, Consultant Radiologist, MRI Unit, St George's Hospital, London, for reading the section on principles of magnetic resonance, and that of my wife Catriona Woodruff for preparing the figures and for help with the manuscript.

References

(1) Lauterbur PC. Image formation of induced local interactions: examples employing NMR. *Nature* 1973; 242: 190–1.
(2) Hollister LE, Boutros N. Clinical use of CT and MR scans in psychiatric patients. *J Psychiat Neurosci* 1991; 16(4): 194–8.
(3) Jack CR, Gehring DG, Sharbrough FW et al. Temporal lobe volume measurement from MR images: accuracy and left–right asymmetry in normal persons. *J Comp Ass Tomog* 1988; 12: 21–9.
(4) Bear D, Schiff D, Saver J, Greenberg M, Freeman R. Quantitative analysis of cerebral asymmetries. *Arch Neurol* 1986; 43: 598–603.
(5) De Lacoste-Utamsing C, Holloway RL. Sexual dimorphism in the human corpus callosum. *Science* 1982; 216: 1431–2.
(6) Witelson SF. Hand and sex differences in the isthmus and genu of the human corpus callosum. *Brain* 1989; 112: 799–833.
(7) Kertesz A, Black SE, Polk M, Howell J. Cerebral asymmetries on magnetic resonance imaging. *Cortex* 1986; 22: 117–27.
(8) Andreason NC, Nasrallah HA, Dunn V et al. Structural abnormalities in the frontal system in schizophrenia. *Arch Gen Psychiat* 1986; 43: 137–44.
(9) Jernigan TL, Press GA, Hesselink JR. Methods for measuring brain morphologic features on magnetic resonance images, validation and normal aging. *Arch Neurol* 1990; 47: 27–32.
(10) Jernigan TL, Archibald SL, Berhow MT, Sowell ER, Foster DS, Hesselink JR. Cerebral structure on MRI, Part I: localization of age-related changes. *Biol Psychiat* 1991; 29: 55–67.
(11) Murphy DGM, DeCarli C, Schapiro MB, Rapoport SI, Horwitz B. Age-related differences in volumes of subcortical nuclei, brain matter, and

cerebrospinal fluid in healthy men as measured with magnetic resonance imaging. *Arch Neurol* 1992; 49: 839–45.
(12) Lim KO, Zipursky RB, Murphy GM, Pfefferbaum A. In vivo quantification of the limbic system using MRI: effects of normal aging. *Psychiat Res: Neuroimaging* 1990; 35: 15–26.
(13) Pearlson GD, Kim WS, Kubos KL et al. Ventricle–brain ratio, computed tomographic density, and brain area in 50 schizophrenics. *Arch Gen Psychiat* 1989; 46: 690–7.
(14) Andreasen NC, Flaum M, Swayze V et al. Intelligence and brain structure in normal individuals. *Am J Psychiat* 1993; 150(1): 130–4.
(15) Andreasen NC, Erhardt JC, Swayze VW et al. Magnetic resonance imaging of the brain in schizophrenia: the pathophysiologic significance of structural abnormalities. *Arch Gen Psychiat* 1990; 47: 35–44.
(16) Ross HE, Glaser FB, Germanson T. The prevalence of psychiatric disorders in patients with alcohol and other drug problems. *Arch Gen Psychiat* 1988; 45: 1023–31.
(17) Bernadt M, Murray RM. Psychiatric disorder, drinking and alcoholism, what are the links? *Br J Psychiat* 1986; 148: 393–400.
(18) Gurling HMD, Curtis D, Murray RM. Psychological deficit from excessive alcohol consumption: evidence from a co-twin control study. *Br J Addict* 1991; 86: 151–5.
(19) Harper CG, Kril JJ. Neuropathology of alcoholism. *Alcohol Alcoholism* 1990; 25: 207–16.
(20) Mann K, Batra A, Gunthner A, Schroth G. Do women develop alcoholic brain damage more readily than men? *Alcoholism: Clin Exp Res* 1992; 16(6): 1052–6.
(21) Jensen GB, Pakkenberg B. Do alcoholics drink their neurones away? *Lancet* 1993; 342: 1201–4.
(22) Zipursky RB, Lim KO, Sullivan EV. Widespread cerebral grey matter volume in schizophrenia. *Arch Gen Psychiat* 1992; 49(3): 195–205.
(23) Chick JD, Smith MA, Engleman HM et al. Magnetic resonance imaging of the brain in alcoholics: cerebral atrophy, lifetime alcohol consumption, and cognitive deficits. *Alcoholism: Clin Exp Res* 1989; 13: 512–18.
(24) Jernigan TL, Butters N, DiTraglia G et al. Reduced cerebral grey matter observed in alcoholics using magnetic resonance imaging. *Alcoholism: Clin Exp Res* 1991; 15(3): 418–27.
(25) Pfefferbaum A, Lim KO, Zipursky RB et al. Brain gray and white matter volume loss accelerates with aging in chronic alcoholics: a quantitive MRI study. *Alcoholism: Clin Exp Res* 1992; 16(6): 1078–89.
(26) Strang J, Gurling H. Computerized tomography and neuropsychological assessment in long-term high-dose heroin addicts. *Br J Addict* 1989; 84: 1011–19.
(27) Leira HL, Myhr G, Nilsen G, Dale LG. Cerebral magnetic resonance imaging and cerebral computerized tomography for patients with solvent-induced encephalopathy. *Scand J Work, Environm Health* 1992; 18(2): 68–70.
(28) Schmauss C, Krieg JC. Enlargement of cerebrospinal fluid spaces in long-term benzodiazephine abusers. *Psych Med* 1987; 17: 869–73.
(29) Suddath RL, Christison GW, Torrey EF, Casanova MF, Weinberger DR.

Anatomical abnormalities in the brains of monozygotic twins discordant for schizophrenia. *New Engl J Med* 1990; 322: 789–94.
(30) Coffey CE, Weiner RD, Djang WT et al. Brain anatomic effects of electroconvulsive therapy. *Arch Gen Psychiat* 1991; 48: 1013–21.
(31) Mander AJ, Whitfield A, Kean DM et al. Cerebral and brain stem changes after ECT revealed by nuclear magnetic resonance imaging. *Br J Psychiat* 1987; 151: 69–71.
(32) Degreef G, Ashtari M, Bogerts B et al. Volumes of ventricular system subdivisions measured from magnetic resonance images in first-episode schizophrenic patients. *Arch Gen Psychiat* 1992; 49: 531–7.
(33) Arndt S, Cohen G, Alliger RJ et al. Problems with ratio and proportion measures of imaged cerebral structures. *J Psychiat Res: Neuroimaging* 1991; 40(1): 79–89.
(34) Kelsoe JR, Cadet JL, Pickar D, Weinberger DR. Quantitative neuroanatomy in schizophrenia. *Arch Gen Psychiat* 1988; 45: 533–41.
(35) Young AH, Blackwood DHR, Roxborough H, McQueen JK, Martin MJ, Kean D. A magnetic resonance imaging study of schizophrenia: brain structure and clinical symptoms. *Br J Psychiat* 1991; 158: 158–64.
(36) Johnstone EC, Owens DGC, Crow TJ et al. Temporal lobe structure as determined by nuclear magnetic resonance in schizophrenia and bipolar affective disorder. *J Neurosurg Psychiat* 1989; 52: 736–41.
(37) Barta PE, Pearlson GD, Powers RE, Richards SS. Tune LE. Auditory hallucinations and smaller superior temporal gyral volume in schizophrenia. *Am J Psychiat* 1990; 147: 1457–62.
(38) Shenton ME, Kikinis R. Jolesz FA et al. Left-lateralized temporal lobe abnormalities in schizophrenia and their relationship to thought disorder. A computerized, quantitive MRI study. *New Engl J Med* 1992; 327: 604–12.
(39) Harvey I, Ron MA, DuBoulay G, Wicks D, Lewis SW, Murray RM. Reduction of cortical volume in schizophrenia on magnetic resonance imaging. *Psych Med* 1993; 23: 591–604.
(40) Woodruff PWR, Pearlson GD, Geer MJ, Barta PE, Chilcoat HD. A computerized magnetic resonance imaging study of corpus callosum morphology in schizophrenia. *Psych Med* 1993; 23: 45–56.
(41) Goldberg TE, Raglan JD, Torrey EF, Gold JM, Bigelow LB, Weinberger DR. Neuropsychological assessment of monozygotic twins discordant for schizophrenia. *Arch Gen Psychiat* 1990; 47: 1066–72.
(42) Weinberger DR, Berman KF, Suddath R, Torrey EF. Evidence of dysfunction of a prefrontal–limbic network in schizophrenia: a magnetic resonance imaging and regional cerebral blood flow study of discordant monozygotic twins. *Am J Psychiat* 1992; 149: 880–97.
(43) Breier A, Buchanan RW, Elkashef A, Munson RC, Kirkpatrick B, Gellad F. A magnetic resonance imaging study of limbic, prefrontal cortex, and caudate structures. *Arch Gen Psychiat* 1992; 49: 921–5.
(44) Woodruff PWR, Howard R, Rushe T, Graves M, Murray RM. Frontal lobe volume and cognitive estimation in schizophrenia. *Schizophrenia Res* 1994 (in press).
(45) Williamson P, Pelz D, Merskey H, Morrison S, Conlon P. Correlation of

negative symptoms in schizophrenia with frontal lobe parameters on magnetic resonance imaging. *Br J Psychiat* 1991; 159: 130–4.

(46) DeLisi LE, Stritzke P, Riordan H et al. The timing of brain morphological changes in schizophrenia and their relationship to clinical outcome. *Biol Psychiat* 1992; 31: 241–54.

(47) Bogerts B, Ashtari M, Degreef G, Alvir JMJ, Bilder RM, Lieberman JA. Reduced temporal limbic structure volumes on magnetic resonance images in first episode schizophrenia. *Psychiat Res: Neuroimaging* 1990; 35: 1–13.

(48) Rossi A, Stratta P, D'Albenzio et al. Reduced temporal lobe areas in schizophrenia. Preliminary evidence from a controlled multi-planar magnetic resonance imaging study. *Biol Psychiat* 1990; 27: 61–8.

(49) Dauphinais D, DeLisi LE, Crow TJ et al. Reduction in temporal lobe size in siblings with schizophrenia: a magnetic resonance imaging study. *Psychiat Res* 1990; 35: 137–47.

(50) Rossi A, Stratta P, Mattei P et al. Planum temporale in schizophrenia: a magnetic resonance study. *Schizophrenia Res* 1992; 7: 19–22.

(51) Jernigan TL, Zisook S, Heaton RK et al. Magnetic resonance imaging abnormalities in lenticular nuclei and cerebral cortex in schizophrenia. *Arch Gen Psychiat* 1991; 48(10): 881–90.

(52) David AS. Tachistoscopic tests of colour naming and matching in schizophrenia: evidence for posterior callosal dysfunction? *Psych Med* 1987; 17: 621–30.

(53) Coger RW, Serafetinides EA. Schizophrenia, corpus callosum, and inter-hemispheric communication: a review. *Psychiat Res* 1990; 34: 163–84.

(54) Lewis SW, Reveley MA, David AS, Ron MA. Agenesis of the corpus callosum and schizophrenia: a case report. *Psych Med* 1988; 18: 341–7.

(55) Swayze W, Andreasen NC, Erhardt JC, Yuh WTC, Allinger RJ, Cohen GA. Development abnormalities of the corpus callosum in schizophrenia: an MRI study. *Arch Neurol* 1990; 47: 805–8.

(56) Lewis SW, Mezey GC. Clinical correlates of septum pellucidum cavities: an unusual association with psychosis. *Psych Med* 1985; 15: 43–54.

(57) Bigelow LB, Nasrallah HA, Rauscher FP. Corpus callosum thickness in chronic schizophrenia. *Br J Psychiat* 1983; 142: 284–7.

(58) Nasrallah HA, Andreasen NC, Coffman JA et al. A controlled magnetic resonance imaging study of corpus callosum thickness in schizophrenia. *Biol Psychiat* 1986; 21: 274–82.

(59) Raine A, Harrison GN, Reynolds GP, Sheard C, Cooper JE, Medley I. Structural and functional characteristics of the corpus callosum in schizophrenics, psychiatric controls, and normal controls. *Arch Gen Psychiat* 1990; 47: 1060–3.

(60) Gunther W, Petsch R, Steinberg R et al. Brain dysfunction during motor activation and corpus callosum alterations in schizophrenia measured by cerebral blood flow and magnetic resonance imaging. *Biol Psychiat* 1991; 29: 535–53.

(61) Casanova MF, Sanders RD, Goldberg TE et al. Morphometry of the corpus callosum in monozygotic twins discordant for schizophrenia: a magnetic resonance imaging study. *J Neurol, Neurosurg Psychiat* 1990; 53: 416–21.

(62) McDonald WM, Krishnan KRR. Magnetic resonance in patients with affective illness. *Eur Arch Psychiat Clin Neurosci* 1992; 241: 283–90.
(63) Altshuler LL, Conrad A, Hauser P et al. Reduction of temporal lobe volume in bipolar disorder: a preliminary report of magnetic resonance imaging. *Arch Gen Psychiat* 1991; 48: 482–3.
(64) Coffey CE, Wilkinson WE, Weiner RD et al. Quantitative cerebral anatomy in depression: a controlled magnetic resonance imaging study. *Arch Gen Psychiat* 1993; 50: 7–16.
(65) Coffman JA, Bornstein RA, Olson SC, Schwarzkopf SB, Nasrallah HA. Cognitive impairment and cerebral structure by MRI in bipolar disorder. *Biol Psychiat* 1990; 27: 1188–96.
(66) Krishnan KRR, McDonald WM, Escalona PR et al. Magnetic resonance imaging of the caudate nuclei in depression. *Arch Gen Psychiat* 1992; 49: 553–7.
(67) Shah SA, Doraiswamy PM, Husain M et al. Posterior fossa abnormalities in major depression: a controlled magnetic resonance imaging study. *Acta Psychiat Scand* 1992; 85(6): 474–9.
(68) Krishnan KRR, Goli V, Ellinwood EH, France RK, Blazer DG, Nemeroff CB. Leukoencephalopathy in patients diagnosed as major depressive. *Biol Psychiat* 1988; 23: 519–22.
(69) Coffey CE, Djang WT, Weiner RD. Subcortical hyperintensities on MRI: a comparison of normal and depressed elderly subjects. *Am J Psychiat* 1990; 147: 187–9.
(70) Figiel GS, Krishnan KRR, Doraiswamy PM, Rao VP, Nemeroff CB, Boyko OB. Subcortical hyperintensities on brain magnetic resonance imaging: a comparison between late age onset and early onset elderly depressed subjects. *Neurobiol Aging* 1991; 26: 245–7.
(71) Coffey CE, Weiner RD, Djang WT et al. Brain anatomic effects of electroconsulsive therapy: a prospective magnetic resonance imaging study. *Arch Gen Psychiat* 1991; 48: 1013–21.

Structural and functional endophenotypes in schizophrenia

T SHARMA

Introduction

Schizophrenia is a common disorder that is likely to consist of a heterogeneous collection of subtypes. Family, twin and adoption studies have established the role of genetics in the aetiology of schizophrenia[1,2]. Genetic analyses have estimated that from 66% to 93% of the variance in the aetiology of schizophrenia is genetic in origin[3–7]. The possibility of genetic heterogeneity is increasingly likely and although Mendelian patterns of inheritance seem to occur in some families, no convincing evidence of specific linkage has been shown[2]. Current evidence also suggests that the offspring of MZ twins discordant for schizophrenia are at greatly increased risk for developing schizophrenia irrespective of whether they are the offspring of the affected or unaffected twin[8]. Unfortunately, genetic family studies have been unable to identify homogeneous subtypes of schizophrenia with the use of clinical criteria. Reviewers of genetic linkage and segregation analysis in schizophrenia have supported the search for genetic susceptibility through the study of biological vulnerability traits and genetic markers[9].

Strong evidence also exists from genetic epidemiological studies of schizophrenia that what is transmitted in families includes the liability to such features as poor psychosocial functioning, suspiciousness and oddness as well as to psychotic illness. Indeed, most studies have found a higher risk of schizophrenia spectrum disorders in the relatives of schizophrenic patients than in the relatives of controls[1]. These abnormalities are likely to be due to the genetic vulnerability to develop schizophrenia and thus have a much higher prevalence in patients with schizophrenia and their family members.

Biological markers which segregate with the disease and are also evident in unaffected family members would increase the power of genetic linkage

All correspondence to: Dr T Sharma, Institute of Psychiatry, De Crespigny Park, Denmark Hill, London SE5 8AF, UK.

Cambridge Medical Reviews: Neurobiology and Psychiatry Volume 3

analysis by identifying phenocopies, classifying asymptomatic cases, increasing penetrance and the selecting homogeneous subgroups. This would then provide a more accurate knowledge of the mode of inheritance. The phenotypic expression of schizophrenia depends on the genetic vulnerability (which is deemed necessary) and independent or interactive environmental insults that finally lead to the overt expression of the disorder[2,8]. These vulnerability markers are more likely to be expressed as they are closer to the gene action and thus more penetrant. Rieder and Gershon[10] have proposed certain criteria for identification of vulnerability markers. These include longitudinal stability, sensitivity and specificity of expression with respect to the target disorder, and a relative insensitivity with respect to co-variates such as gender, age, medication status, social class and clinical state effects.

Major research effort over the past decade has gone into looking for biological or behavioural characteristics in schizophrenia patients and their first-degree relatives, using event-related brain potentials (mainly P300), eye tracking, neuropsychology and structural brain imaging. Investigators have used designs that look for these markers in identical twins discordant for schizophrenia, and siblings and parents of schizophrenia patients as well as children at high risk where one or both parents suffer from schizophrenia. Some of the studies carried out in search of such biological markers in first-degree relatives of schizophrenia patients will be selectively reviewed in this chapter.

Studies of putative electrophysiological and neuropsychological markers

Family members of patients with schizophrenia have been reported to be more likely than controls to show poor performance of complex motor tasks[11], on cognitive tests such as the Wisconsin Card Sorting Test[12], exhibit abnormal eye movements and prolonged event-related brain potentials[13]. Such 'endophenotypic' markers in these individuals with genetic loading for schizophrenia may point towards an underlying phenotype that is not expressed clinically. Ultimately, this may help in identifying the genetic and environmental contributions to the aetiology of schizophrenia.

Event-related brain potentials

Studies of event-related brain potentials (ERP) using the 'oddball' paradigm have mainly reported on the auditory P300 response (a positive deflection elicited 300 ms after the stimulus). The latency of the auditory P300 response has high concordance in normal monozygotic (MZ) twin pairs[14,14a]. Schizophrenia patients show reduced amplitude and increased latency of the P300 wave, but this characteristic is not specific to schizophrenia as similar variations are also seen in alcoholism, dementia, major depression and schizotypal disorder[15–17]. P300 latency appears to be independent of the effects of medication and the clinical state at the time of testing[16]. Kidogami et al[18] found decreased amplitude while Blackwood et al[13] reported increased latency in siblings and parents of schizophrenic probands. Schreiber et al[19–21] reported prolonged P300 latencies in children at high risk of schizophrenia compared with age, sex and education matched controls. Frangou et al[22] reported a bimodal distribution in the P300 latency in the unaffected first-degree relatives in multiply affected families suggesting that some of the unaffected relatives were possible carriers of the schizophrenia genotype. This finding, which replicates the study by Blackwood et al[13], points towards a brain disturbance possibly linked to the development of schizophrenia in the probands of these families.

Neuropsychology

Neuropsychological assessments in relatives of schizophrenia patients have shown deficits in sustained attention, perceptual–motor speed, concept formation, abstraction and to a lesser extent on mental control and encoding. Verbal memory and verbal fluency impairments have also been found in schizophrenics and their first-degree relatives[23,24]. A subgroup of children of schizophrenic parents, when compared with children of normal parents, have been shown to exhibit impairment on test of attention, learning, verbal ability and neuromotor functions[23]. This supports the notion that this subgroup of children may have inherited the liability to develop schizophrenia later in life, and this liability is being exhibited as cognitive and motor impairments in their childhood. Studies of siblings of schizophrenia patients have also shown impairment in sustained attention, abstraction and language function[25–28]. Cannon et al[26] have shown that the pattern of deficits are similar in schizophrenic probands and their relatives, thus suggesting dysfunction in the prefrontal, temporo-limbic and attentional circuits. The performance of the non-schizophrenic siblings was intermediate between that of the schizophrenic siblings and the normal controls on all measures of functioning on a comprehensive neuropsychological test battery. The shapes of the deficit profiles were similar in the probands and the siblings with 80% of the probands showing more deviant scores than their siblings. Verbal memory, abstraction, attention and language function were impaired in the schizophrenic probands and their siblings in this study. Goldberg et al[29] applied the twin paradigm to test the effect of genetic factors on neuropsychological profiles in discordant MZ twins. Though they did not find any statistical significant differences between the non-schizophrenic twins and the normal twins, the well twins' scores were deviant in most of the comparisons carried out. The presence of abnormalities in unaffected relatives of schizophrenic probands rules out confounding effects of the illness process and subsequent treatment.

Eye tracking

Investigators have used two main types of eye tracking to study eye tracking abnormalities in schizophrenia patients and their relatives. 'Smooth pursuit' eye movements enable the subject to follow a slowly moving target object and maintain a stable image on the retina. 'Saccadic' eye movements are rapid step-like movements that enable the eye to quickly fix on a target. Antisaccadic eye movements (a variant of the saccadic eye movements) paradigms are also used in assessing eye tracking abnormalities where the subject is asked to look in the opposite direction of the target. These different types of eye movements are controlled by separate neuronal circuits. Neuroleptic medication has very little effect on smooth pursuit eye movements and as abnormalities are also seen in remission they are likely to be trait rather than state markers. The pair-wise concordance rate for eye tracking dysfunction (ETD) in MZ twins discordant for schizophrenia was higher than that found in dizygotic twins discordant for schizophrenia[30–32], suggesting that genetic factors contributed to the variability of smooth pursuit eye movements. ETD in the proband is also associated with ETD in some of the first-degree relatives of the proband[13,30,32–34], but there are reports of patients with good eye tracking who have relatives exhibiting ETD[35].

Post-mortem studies in schizophrenia

An array of structural brain abnormalities have been reported in the literature on neuropathology of schizophrenia. These studies have driven some of the structural neuroimaging studies in schizophrenia. Post-mortem studies have reported decreased size of the hippocampus, decreased white matter in the temporal lobes and parahippocampal gyrus and abnormalities in cellular alignment, loss of normal cerebral asymmetry and cytoarchitectural abnormalities of the superficial layers of the entorhinal cortex[36–45]. Current evidence from neuropathological studies is, therefore, more consistent with the hypothesis that brain abnormalities found in schizophrenia are due to an abnormality in brain development. The lack of gliosis in brains of patients with schizophrenia indicates that there is probably no neuronal damage after the sixth month of gestation[46]. Studies have also reported reduced brain weight by approximately 6%, and an increase in the volume of the lateral ventricles in patients with schizophrenia[47].

Structural brain imaging in schizophrenia

Magnetic resonance imaging (MRI) has replaced computerized tomography (CT) as the structural imaging modality of choice primarily due to its increased resolution and multiplanar capability. Lateral and third ventricular enlargement as well as cortical sulcal enlargement are the most consistent neuroanatomical changes found in schizophrenia[48]. MRI studies have replicated the earlier CT studies but also show an increase in sulcal fluid in the general cortical[49–51], as well as in the frontotemporal and temporoparietal regions[52]. Studies have been driven by the neuropathological literature and reduced temporal lobe volume as well as reduced temporal lobe grey matter have been described by some[53,54], but not others[55,56]. Reduced hippocampal volume in male schizophrenics on MRI scan have now been described by Bogerts et al[57] while Barta et al[58] have described reduced superior temporal gyrus volume and left amygdala volume.

Two recent studies have reported widespread grey matter volume decrements in schizophrenia[52,59]. Zipursky et al[52] reported that grey matter volumes, but not white matter volumes, were significantly reduced in schizophrenics while Harvey et al[59] found a significant decrease in cortical volume and corresponding increase in sulcal fluid. These findings suggest that schizophrenic patients may have significant widespread deficits in grey matter volume and this may underlie the cortical sulcal and ventricular volume increases reported with CT. The finding of reduced grey matter volume in schizophrenia on MRI is also consistent with the gross neuropathological finding of Pakkenburg[60], who found a 12% reduction in cortical grey matter volume in patients with schizophrenia but no significant change in white matter volume. This challenges the supposition that medial limbic structures are the main site of brain pathology in schizophrenia. First-episode MRI studies have also shown abnormalities, thus suggesting that they are not artefacts of treatment or chronicity[61,62].

Structural abnormalities and genetics of schizophrenia

Brain growth is under genetic control, and 30% of humane genes are expressed exclusively in the brain[63]. Raz and Raz[64] reviewed 93 neuroimaging studies and determined that there is a 57% overlap in ventricular size between schizophrenics and controls, thus making ventricular size a poor marker for schizophrenia. This is possibly due to normal genetic variation of brain structure in humans rather than heterogeneous schizophrenic populations as there does not seem to be any prominent correlation of structural abnormalities with chronicity of the illness. Moreover, there is evidence of a unimodal distribution with a positive skew rather than a bimodal distribution of structural brain abnormalities in pooled data. Thus, the problem may be with the control groups chosen. One way of circumventing this problem would be to choose first-degree relatives of family history negative schizophrenic probands as controls. Several investigators have tried to address this issue by choosing their own aetiological models of the illness and then applying a particular study design to answer the hypotheses raised by the model. These studies have tried to tease out the genetic and environmental contributions to brain abnormalities in schizophrenia.

Studies of identical twins discordant for schizophrenia

Reveley et al[65] suggested that ventricular size is under substantial genetic control. They found a high degree of heritability in ventricular size in both normal MZ twins (98%) and in MZ twins discordant for schizophrenia (87%) while normal dizygotic twins showed a heritability of 78%. They studied 11 MZ twin pairs discordant for schizophrenia and reported that the affected twin showed significantly larger ventricles than twins from normal pairs while the unaffected twin showed total ventricular volumes of intermediate value[66]. One interpretation is that a genetic factor contributes to ventricular enlargement in both twins and that environmental injury may have occurred in addition to the underlying genetic liability to further increase ventricular size in the schizophrenic twin. Suddath et al[67], using MRI, studied 15 MZ twins discordant for schizophrenia and reported smaller anterior hippocampi and enlarged lateral and third ventricles in the brains of the schizophrenic twins compared with their well co-twins. The schizophrenic twins also showed a reduction in the volume of the temporal grey matter that was more marked on the left. Furthermore, in 12 of 15 discordant twin pairs in this study, the affected twin could be identified on blind visual inspection of the scans. However, they did not have a comparison group of normal twins to ascertain whether the unaffected twins had any structural brain abnormalities.

Studies of schizophrenic probands and their unaffected siblings and parents

Weinberger et al[68] found that all of the schizophrenic patients had the largest ventricles of their siblings and that the schizophrenic patients had significantly larger ventricles than their siblings and controls. However, the well siblings of the schizophrenic patients also had larger ventricles than controls. Using a similar strategy, DeLisi et al[69] studied the ventricular size of schizophrenic probands from multiply affected families. The patients with schizophrenia had larger ventricles than the controls but were not significantly different from their non-schizophrenic siblings whose mean ventricular size was approximately mid-way in value between the patients' and volunteers' values. Honer et al[70] reported brain abnormalities on MRI in two members of a multiply affected schizophrenic family showing a partial trisomy on chromosome 5. Bilateral temporal lobe atrophy was seen in two affected individuals, and one individual showed evidence of developmental abnormalities, i.e. a cavum septum pellucidum and a cavum vergae.

Studies of high-risk samples where subjects have one or both parents suffering from schizophrenia

Cannon and co-workers proposed the diathesis-stress model as a result of their CT studies in the Copenhagen high-risk sample[71]. It posits that genetic factors interact with environmental factors to produce schizophrenia and its accompanying brain changes. Cannon et al[72] studied 34 high-risk children of schizophrenic mothers from their Copenhagen high-risk sample. Cortical and cerebellar abnormalities were predicted by the presence of schizophrenia spectrum disorder (the only additional genetic variance) in the father but not related to pregnancy or birth events while third and lateral ventricular enlargement was predicted primarily by the interaction of the genetic risk for schizophrenia and delivery complications. The study design, however, did not allow the investigators to examine the effect of obstetric complications in the absence of genetic risk as all the children had schizophrenic mothers. Thus, there was a proposal that there may be two separate pathways that caused brain abnormalities with genetic factors concentrating mainly on the cortex. In a larger sample from the same high-risk sample, Cannon et al[26] examined 60, 72 and 25 individuals with neither, one or two parents, respectively, who were affected with schizophrenia spectrum disorder. They reported that there was a stepwise linear increase in cortical and ventricular cerebrospinal fluid–brain ratios on CT scans with increasing level of genetic risk for schizophrenia. Individuals with two affected parents evidenced greater ventricular and sulcal enlargement than those with one affected parent, who in turn evidenced greater ventricular enlargement than those with no affected parents. They conclude that the type and degree of brain abnormalities shown by adult offspring of schizophrenic and normal parents are predicted by the independent and interacting influences of genetic risk for schizophrenia and obstetric complications.

Studies of schizophrenics compared on the basis of family history and environmental insults

The familial–non-familial hypothesis proposed by Murray and colleagues[73] has been the cornerstone of studies assessing schizophrenic probands on the basis of family history. The hypothesis posits that genetic predisposition itself can lead to the development of schizophrenia when there is high genetic loading. In the presence of low genetic predisposition, environmental factors are required to produce schizophrenia in a predisposed individual. Lewis et al[73] have applied their hypothesis to brain structure and have proposed that patients who develop schizophrenia on a genetic basis will not have structural brain changes, whereas those with sporadic cases may have a structural brain abnormality to account for their developing schizophrenia[66]. However, the relationship between brain scan appearance and family history of schizophrenia has been a subject of controversy. Many have found no difference in CT scans between those with and those without a positive family history[74]. Others have reported significant results but the direction of the relationship has varied, with some finding larger lateral ventricles in the non-familial disorders[66,75,76] and some demonstrating the reverse[77]. Thus, this hypothesis has been subjected to theoretical criticism and fails to account completely for the occasional reports of brain scan abnormalities in familial schizophrenia. Lewis[78] later reviewed the studies up to 1990 that addressed this issue and concluded that the hypothesis that ventricular enlargement was confined to those without a family history of mental illness is now 'outdated'. Of the 13 studies reviewed by Lewis, three found a significant inverse correlation between ventricular size and positive family history, one found a positive correlation, one found a curvilinear association and the remaining studies found no relationship. One explanation for these discrepancies would be that a positive family history of schizophrenia is associated with a moderate rather than a major degree of ventricular enlargement. Owens et al[79] described a complex curvilinear relationship between family history and ventricle–brain ratio (VBR); the highest frequency of positive family history scores occurred in those with medium VBRs. In any comparison between family history positive and family history negative schizophrenics, the pattern of differences will depend not only on the brain scan appearances of the familial patients but also on the composition of the remaining patient sample. Roy and Crowe[80] have recently reviewed the literature and found little support for any strong association between brain abnormalities and presence or absence of family history of schizophrenia. They used a scale that assessed 10 methodological features in each study and included those studies that achieved a minimum score of 50% of their total score. Their criteria were fairly rigorous and they included six CT and two MRI studies in their review. Whenever a difference was reported in these studies, between familial and sporadic schizophrenics, the familial schizophrenics had the more extreme abnormalities, suggesting that structural abnormalities may reflect genetic factors.

The evidence from CT and MRI studies suggests that genetic risk for schizophrenia may be a determinant of the cortical abnormalities reported in schizophrenia. While MZ twin studies have informed us about the possible non-genetic contribution to structural brain abnormalities in schizophrenia, high-risk and family studies show that structural brain abnormalities tend to aggregate in families and is partly under genetic control as the pathology increases linearly with the number of affected relatives. This raises the possibility that the structural abnormalities found in the brains of patients with schizophrenia may be due to a genetically determined developmental abnormality that might also be present to some extent in those family members carrying the same genetic vulnerability.

Methodological problems encountered in structural brain imaging studies

These studies, however, have not been consistent in controlling rigorously for confounding variables in the interpretation of brain size. Some of these confounders are the effects of age, handedness, parental socioeconomic class, ethnicity, genetic loading, differences in intracranial volume or the possibility that other brain regions may show similar effects[52,81,82]. Variable inclusion and exclusion criteria (differences in demographic characteristics, age, sex and ethnicity) reduce the strength of the studies[78]. The screening of normal controls and the use of neurological patients or medical patients as controls when their scans had been passed as 'normal' by a radiologist, is another drawback. The methodological weakness of the family history method has been in the definition of family history where the subjects were assigned to groups based on their own reports of family history or reports of informants, without interviewing the other first-degree relatives. False negatives are likely to be due to small family size or systematic evasion of the diagnostic process[69]. False positives are likely when family history is defined as presence of any psychiatric disorder in first- or second-degree relatives of the proband. Some investigators[83] have relied on case notes to classify individuals on family history.

Conclusions

The search for endophenotypes has resulted in interesting positive findings for investigators looking for a genetic contribution to the inheritance of these biological markers. However, these reports are tempered by the fact that there are limitations to the interpretation of statistical differences in these studies in the absence of normative data. There are no studies in normal families to look at the heritability of these markers though some twin studies have been carried out. The effect of confounding variables that may contribute to false positive results needs to be taken into account, e.g. the effect of age on these variables when parents of probands are included as first-degree relatives in family studies. The specificity of these markers have not yet been fully established as there are no comparisons with families of affective disorder probands. The sensitivity of these markers as indicators of schizophrenia needs to be established by carrying out within-family comparisons. ERPs do not seem to have diagnostic specificity and there is overreliance on the oddball paradigm. The most important gap in the structural imaging literature is an obvious one: there is no normative data on the variation of the brain structure with respect to sex, age, ethnicity, education and family affiliation for the populations being studied. Without this data assumptions will be made about the control and affected groups based on very little hard evidence. A probabilistic brain atlas would go a long way towards disentangling these variables.

References

(1) Kendler KS. The genetics of schizophrenia and related disorders: a review. In: Dunner DL, Gershon ES, Barrett JE, eds. *Relatives at risk for mental disorder*. New York: Raven Press Ltd; 1988.

(2) Gottesman II. *Schizophrenia genesis: the origins of madness*. New York: WH Freeman and Company; 1990: 296.
(3) Fulker DW. A biometrical genetic approach to intelligence and schizophrenia. *Social Biol* 1973; 20: 266–75.
(4) McGue M, Gottesman II, Rao DC. The transmission of schizophrenia under a multifactorial threshold model. *Am J Hum Genet* 1983; 35: 1161–78.
(5) McGue H, Gottesman II, Rao DC. Resolving genetic models of the transmission of schizophrenia. *Gen Epidemiol* 1985; 2: 99–110.
(6) Kendler KS. Overview: a current perspective on twin studies of schizophrenia. *Am J Psychiat* 1983; 140: 1413–25.
(7) Rao DC, Morton NE, Gottesman II, Lew R. Path analysis of qualitative data on pairs of relatives: application to schizophrenia. *Hum Hered* 1981; 31: 325–33.
(8) Gottesman II, Bertelsen A. Confirming unexpressed genotypes for schizophrenia. *Arch Gen Psychiat* 1989; 46: 867–72.
(9) Kendler K. The feasibility of linkage studies in schizophrenia. Dahlem Konferenzen, Biological Perspectives in Schizophrenia, Dahlem Foundation, Wallostr. 10, 1000 Berlin 33; 1986.
(10) Rieder RO, Gershon ES. Genetic strategies in biological psychiatry. *Arch Gen Psychiat* 1978; 35: 866–73.
(11) Griffiths TD, Birkett PBL, Frangou S et al. Neurological signs in patients with familial schizophrenia and their relatives. *Schizophrenia Res* 1994; 11: 194.
(12) Pogue-Geile MF, Garrett AH, Brunke JJ, Hall JK. Neuropsychological impairments are increased in siblings of schizophrenic patients. *Schizophrenia Res* 1991; 4: 390.
(13) Blackwood DG, St Clair DM, Muir WJ, Duffy JC. Auditory P300 and eye tracking dysfunction in schizophrenic pedigrees. *Arch Gen Psychiat* 1991; 48: 899–909.
(14) Surwillo WW. Cortical evoked potentials in monozygotic twins and unrelated subjects: comparisons of exogenous and endogenous components. *Behav Genet* 1980; 10: 201–9.
(14a) Polich J, Burns T. P300 from identical twins. *Neuropsychologia* 1987; 25: 299–304.
(15) Blackwood DH, St Clair DM, Kutcher SP. P300 event-related potential abnormalities in borderline personality disorder. *Biol Psychiat* 1986; 21: 560–4.
(16) Blackwood DHR, Whalley LJ, Christie JE, Blackburn IM, St Clair DM, McInnes A. Changes in auditory P3 event-related potential in schizophrenia and depression. *Biol Psychiat* 1987; 150: 154–60.
(17) Pfefferbaum A, Wenegrat BG, Ford JM, Roth WT. Clinical application of the P3 component of event-related potentials. II. Dementia, depression and schizophrenia. *Electroencephalogr Clin Neurophysiol* 1984; 59: 104–24.
(18) Kidogami Y, Yoneda H, Asaba H, Sakai T. P300 in first degree relatives of schizophrenics. *Schizophrenia Res* 1991; 6: 9–13.
(19) Schreiber H, Stolz G, Rotmeier J, Kornhuber HH, Born J. Prolonged latencies of the N2 and P3 of the auditory event-related potential in children at risk for

schizophrenia. A preliminary report. *Eur Arch Psychiat Neurol Sci* 1989; 238: 185–8.
(20) Schreiber H, Stolz-Born G, Rothmeier J, Kornhuber A, Kornhuber HH, Born J. Endogenous event-related brain potentials and psychometric performance in children at risk for schizophrenia. *Biol Psychiat* 1991; 30: 177–89.
(21) Schreiber H, Stolz-Born G, Kornhuber HH, Born J. Event-related potential correlates of impaired selective attention in children at high risk for schizophrenia. *Biol Psychiat* 1992; 32: 634–51.
(22) Frangou S, Alarcon G, Sharma T, Takei N, Binnie C, Murray RM. P300 in failial and nonfamilial schizophrenia. *Schizophrenia Res* 1994; 11: 159.
(23) Kremen WS, Seidman LJ, Pepple J, Lyons M, Tsuang MT, Faraone SV. Neuropsychological risk indicators for schizophrenia: a review of family studies. *Schizophrenia Bull* 20: 103–20.
(24) Sharma T, Mockler DM, Riordan JM, Davis N. Memory impairment and clinical symptoms in schizophrenia. *Schizophrenia Res* 1994; 11: 186.
(25) Birkett PBL, Sigmundsson T, Sharma T et al. Neuropsychological abnormalities in the relatives of familial schizophrenics. *Schizophrenia Res* 1994; 11: 158.
(26) Cannon TD, Mednick SA, Parnas J, Schulsinger F, Praestholm J, Vestergaard A. Developmental brain abnormalities in the offspring of schizophrenic mothers. *Arch Gen Psychiat* 1993; 50: 551–63.
(27) Mirsky AF, Lochhead SJ, Jones BP, Kugelmass S, Walsh D, Kendler KS. On familial factors in the attentional deficit in schizophrenia: a review and report of two new subject samples. *J Psychiat Res* 1992; 26: 383–403.
(28) Pogue-Geile MF. Siblings of schizophrenic probands: presence of neuropsychological impairments. *Schizophrenia Res* 1990; 3: 62.
(29) Goldberg TE, Ragland JD, Torrey EF, Gold JM, Bigelow LB, Weinberger DR. Neuropsychological assessment of monozygotic twins discordant for schizophrenia. *Arch Gen Psychiat* 1990; 47: 1066–72.
(30) Holzman PS, Kringlen E, Levy DL, Proctor LR, Haberman SJ, Yasillo NJ. Abnormal-pursuit eye movements in schizophrenia. Evidence for a genetic indicator. *Arch Gen Psychiat* 1977; 34: 802–5.
(31) Holzman PS, Kringlen E, Levy DL, Proctor LR, Haberman SJ, Yasillo NJ. Smooth pursuit eye movements in twins discordant for schizophrenia. *J Psychiat Res* 1978; 14: 111–20.
(32) Holzman PS, Kringlen E, Levy DL, Haberman SJ. Deviant eye tracking in twins discordant for psychosis: a replication. *Arch Gen Psychiat* 1980; 37: 627–31.
(33) Holzman PS, Solomon CM, Levin S, Waternaux CS. Pursuit eye movement dysfunctions in schizophrenia. Family evidence for specificity. *Arch Gen Psychiat* 1984; 41: 136–9.
(34) Holzman PS, Levy DL. Smooth pursuit eye movements and functional psychoses; a review. *Schizophrenia Bull* 1977; 3: 15–27.
(35) Iacono WG, Moreau M, Beiser M, Fleming JA, Lin TY. Smooth-pursuit eye tracking in first episode psychotic patients and their relatives. *J Abnormal Psychol* 1992; 101: 104–16.
(36) Benes FM, Bird ED. An analysis of the arrangement of neurons in the

cingulate cortex of schizophrenic patients. *Arch Gen Psychiat* 1987; 33: 608–16.
(37) Benes FM, Davidson J, Bird ED. Quantitative cytoarchitectural studies of the cerebral cortex of schizophrenics. *Arch Gen Psychiat* 43: 31–5.
(38) Benes FM, Majocha R, Bird ED et al. Increased vertical axon numbers in cingulate cortex of schizophrenics. *Arch Gen Psychiat* 1987; 44: 1017–21.
(39) Benes FM, McSparren J, Bird ED et al. Deficits in small interneurons in prefrontal and cingulate cortices of schizophrenic and schizoaffective patients. *Arch Gen Psychiat* 1991; 48: 996–1001.
(40) Bogerts B, Meertz E, Schonfeldt-Bausch R. Basal ganglia and limbic system pathology in schizophrenia. *Arch Gen Psychiat* 1985; 42: 784–91.
(41) Brown R, Colter N, Corsellis JAN et al. Post mortem evidence of structural brain changes in schizophrenia. *Arch Gen Psychiat 1986;* 43: 36–42.
(42) Colter N, Battal S, Crow TJ et al. White matter reduction in the parahippocampal gyrus of patients with schizophrenia (letter). *Arch Gen Psychiat* 1987; 44: 1023.
(43) Jakob H, Beckmann H. Gross and histological criteria for developmental disorders in brains of schizophrenics. *J Roy Soc Med* 1989; 82: 466–9.
(44) Kovelman JA, Scheibel AB. A neurohistological correlate of schizophrenia. *Biol Psychiat* 1984; 19: 1601–21.
(45) Stevens JR. Neuropathology of schizophrenia. *Arch Gen Psychiat* 1982; 39: 1131–9.
(46) Roberts GW. Schizophrenia: the cellular biology of a functional psychosis. *J Neurosci* 1990; 13(6): 207–11.
(47) Bogerts B. Recent advances in the neuropathology of schizophrenia. *Schizophrenia Bull* 1993; 19: 431–5.
(48) Zigun J, Weinberger DR. In vivo studies of brain morphology in patients with schizophrenia. In: Lindenmayer J-P, Kay SR, eds. *New biological vistas on schizophrenia.* New York: Brunner/Mazel; 1992.
(49) Gur RE, Mozley PD, Resnick SM et al. Magnetic resonance imaging in schizophrenia. I. Volumetric analysis of brain and cerebrospinal fluid. *Arch Gen Psychiat* 1991; 48: 407–12.
(50) Jernigan TL, Zisook S, Heaton RK, Moranville JT, Hesselink JR, Braff DL. Magnetic resonance imaging abnormalities in lenticular nuclei and cerebral cortex in schizophrenia. *Arch Gen Psychiat* 1991; 48: 881–90.
(51) Pearlson GD, Marsh L. Magnetic resonance imaging in psychiatry. In: Andreasen NC, section ed., Oldham J, Riba M, Tasman A, eds. *Brain imaging.* Washington, DC: American Psychiatry Press Review of Psychiatry; 1993: 347–82.
(52) Zipursky RB, Lim KO, Sullivan EV, Brown BW, Pfefferbaum A. Widespread cerebral gray matter volume deficits in schizophrenia. *Arch Gen Psychiat* 1992; 49: 195–205.
(53) Suddath R, Casanova MF, Goldberg TE, Daniel DG, Kelsoe JR, Weinberger DR. Temporal lobe pathology in schizophrenia. *Am J Psychiat* 1989; 146: 464–72.
(54) Shenton ME, Kikinis R, Jolesz FA et al. Abnormalities of the left temporal lobe and thought disorder in schizophrenia. A quantitative magnetic resonance imaging study. *N Engl J Med* 1992; 327: 604–12.

(55) Johnstone EC, Owens DG, Crow TJ, Alexandropolis K, Bydder G, Colter N. Temporal lobe structure as determined by nuclear magnetic resonance in schizophrenia and bipolar affective disorder. *J Neurol, Neurosurg Psychiat* 1989; 52: 736–41.

(56) Kelsoe JR, Cadet JL, Pickar D, Weinberger DR. Quantitative neuroanatomy in schizophrenia. *Arch Gen Psychiat* 1988; 45: 533–41.

(57) Bogerts B, Ashtari M, Degreff G, Alvir JM, Bilder RM, Lieberman JA. Reduced temporal limbic structure volumes on magnetic resonance images in first episode schizophrenia. *Psychiat Res* 1990; 35: 1–13.

(58) Barta PE, Pearlson GD, Powers RE, Richards SS, Tune LE. Auditory hallucinations and smaller superior temporal gyral volume in schizophrenia. *Am J Psychiat* 1990; 147: 1457–62.

(59) Harvey I, Ron MA, Du Boulay G, Wicks D, Lewis SW, Murray RM. Reduction of cortical volume in schizophrenia on magnetic resonance imaging. *Psychol Med* 1993; 23: 591–604.

(60) Pakkenberg B. Post-mortem study of chronic schizophrenic brains. *Br J Psychiat* 1987; 151: 744–52.

(61) Degreef G, Ashtari M, Bogerts B et al. Volumes of ventricular system subdivisions measured from magnetic resonance images in first-episode schizophrenic patients. *Arch Gen Psychiat* 1992; 49: 531–7.

(62) DeLisi LE, Stritzke P,. Riordan H et al. The timing of brain morphological changes in schizophrenia and their relationship to clinical outcome. *Biol Psychiat* 1992; 31: 241–54.

(63) Sutcliffe JG, Milner RJ, Gottesfeld JM et al. Control of neuronal gene expression: *Science* 1984; 225: 1308–15.

(64) Raz S, Raz N. Structural brain abnormalities in the major psychoses: a quantitative review of the evidence from computerized imaging. *Psychol Bull* 1990; 108: 93–108.

(65) Reveley AM, Reveley MA, Clifford CA, Murray RM. Cerebral ventricular size in twins discordant for schizophrenia. *Lancet* 1982; i: 540–1.

(66) Reveley AM, Reveley MA, Murray RM. Cerebral ventricular enlargement in non-genetic schizophrenia: a controlled twin study. *Br J Psychiat* 1984; 144: 89–93.

(67) Suddath RL, Christison GW, Torrey EF, Casanova MF, Weinberger DL. Anatomical abnormalities in the brains of monozygotic twins discordant for schizophrenia. *New Engl J Med* 1990; 322: 789–94.

(68) Weinberger DR, DeLisi LE, Neophytides AN, Wyatt RJ. Familial abnormalities in chronic schizophrenic patients. *Psychiat Res* 1981; 4: 65–71.

(69) DeLisi LE, Goldin LR, Hamovit JR, Maxwell ME, Kurtz D, Gershon ES. A family study of the association of increased ventricular size with schizophrenia. *Arch Gen Psychiat* 1986; 43: 148–53.

(70) Honer WG, Bassett AS, MacEwan GW et al. Structural brain imaging abnormalities associated with schizophrenia and partial trisomy of chromosome 5. *Psychol Med* 1992; 22: 519–24.

(71) Cannon TD, Mednick SA, Parnas J. Antecedents of predominantly negative and predominantly positive schizophrenia in a high-risk population. *Arch Gen Psychiat* 1990; 47: 622–32.

(72) Cannon TD, Mednick SA, Parnas J. Genetic and perinatal determinances of structural brain deficits in schizophrenia. *Arch Gen Psychiat* 1989; 46: 833–9.
(73) Lewis SW, Reveley AM, Reveley MA, Chitkara B, Murray RM. The familial/sporadic distinction as a strategy in schizophrenia research. *Br J Psychiat* 1987; 151: 306–13.
(74) Pearlson GD, Garbacz DJ, Moberg PJ. Symptomatic, familial, perinatal and social correlates of computerised axial tomography (CAT) changes in schizophrenics and bipolars. *J Nerv Ment Dis* 1985; 173: 42–50.
(75) Oxenstierna G, Bergstrand G, Bjerkenstedt L. Evidence of disturbed CSF circulation and brain atrophy in cases of schizophrenic psychosis. *Br J Psychiat* 1984; 144: 654–61.
(76) Turner SW, Toone BK, Brett-Jones JR. Computerised tomographic scan changes in early schizophrenia preliminary findings. *Psychol Med* 1986; 16: 219–25.
(77) Nasrallah HA, Kuperman S, Hamra BJ. Clinical differences between schizophrenic patients with and without large cerebral ventricles. *J Clin Psychol* 1983; 44: 407–9.
(78) Lewis SW. Computerized tomography in schizophrenia. 15 years on. *Br J Psychiat* 1990; 157 (suppl): 16–24.
(79) Owens DGS, Johnstone EC, Crow TJ. Lateral ventricular size in schizophrenia: relationship to the disease process and its clinical manifestations. *Psychol Med* 1985; 15: 27–41.
(80) Roy MA, Crowe RR. Validity of the familial and sporadic subtypes of schizophrenia. *Am J Psychiat* 1994; 151: 805–14.
(81) Pfefferbaum A, Lim KO, Rosenbloom M, Zipursky RB. Brain magnetic resonance imaging: approaches for investigating schizophrenia. *Schizophrenia Bull* 1990; 16: 453–76.
(82) Pfefferbaum A, Zipursky RB. Neuroimaging studies of schizophrenia. *Schizophrenia Res* 1991; 4: 193–208.
(83) Schwarzkopf SB, Nasrallah HA, Olson SC, Bogerts B, McLaughlin JA, Mitra T. Family history and brain morphology in schizophrenia: an MRI study. *Psychiat Res* 1991; 40: 49–60.

Techniques for integrating functional and anatomical imaging

H LOATS, S E LOATS and T L RIPPEON

Introduction

Functional and anatomical brain images contain different types of information which play a complementary role in understanding brain function. Differing imaging modalities are generally acquired at different resolutions, scales and aspects. Furthermore, images are stored in various formats. However, 'image fusion' strategies can be used which combine the best features from various imaging modalities.

Positron emission tomography and single-photon emission tomography (PET, SPET) contain functional (physiology-related) information (local glucose metabolism, local protein synthesis, cerebral blood flow, cerebral oxygen utilization, in vivo receptor binding). Differences in the radiolabelled ligands and the acquisition technique for PET and SPET give rise to different capabilities for quantification and biological alteration.

Magnetic resonance imaging and X-ray computed tomographic (MRI, CT) provide relatively high spatial resolution information related to the anatomical and structural aspects of the brain (evidence of structural or anatomical abnormalities or gross tissue pathology). MRI provides good soft-tissue discriminability, while CT provides excellent definition of bony structures, with reduced contrast for soft-tissue.

Images derived from PET and SPET each provide functional information. For each of these imaging modalities, however, the absolute interpretation is compromised significantly by relatively low spatial resolution and variable anatomical specificity. Because of the inherently poor resolution, and due to perturbations caused by varying behavioural patterns, these modalities do not generally present precisely defined or easily perceived anatomical landmarks. MRI and CT, on the other hand, provide

All correspondence to: Dr H Loats, Loats Associates Inc, PO Box 528, Westminster, Maryland 21158, USA.

Cambridge Medical Reviews: Neurobiology and Psychiatry Volume 3

higher spatial resolution with good anatomical landmark visibility, but do not convey physiological functional information.

However, even though the two classes of images (functional and anatomical) provide different information, they have in the past mainly been used in a single-mode fashion. Usually, a single imaging mode is chosen which 'best' satisfies the requirements of diagnostic or research paradigms for specific diseases, conditions or classes of subjects. Currently, comparative review of alternative modalities takes the form of side-by-side visual comparison of slice images. Techniques which simultaneously use complementary information from more than one imaging modality have only recently come into use.

To overcome the shortcomings of the individual imaging modalities, and to answer many important clinical and research questions related to the brain, strategies of computer-graphics generated image fusion can be adopted, which combine the best features of both imaging modalities in a synergistic fashion. Image fusion superimposes the functional information from PET/SPET images on to an anatomical image substrate derived from registered MRI/CT images so that both can be viewed and analysed in a simultaneous fashion. The fusion techniques provide new information based on visual and analytical anatomical–physiological correlation. Anatomically derived regions of interest can be used to quantify the functional 'activity'. Activity peaks, clusters and minimum can be understood from a spatial–anatomical perspective.

The advent, and rapidly increasing growth of fast, low-cost graphics/image-orientated microcomputers has fostered the development of these techniques for fusing (combining) and analysing multimodal volume–brain image data sets. Mathematical image processing techniques and algorithms for registering, merging (fusion) and analysing functional and anatomical images of the brain are currently being developed rapidly. In addition, improved methods for anatomically specific quantitation of cortical surfaces and internal structures of the brain are beginning to be used. Visualization of the functional and anatomical information in a 3D context, previously requiring significant expert mental image transformation, can now be done by image superposition and integration.

Examples of image fusion are: 1) localization of regions in the brain which isolate auditory processing phenomena (combined PET and MRI)[1]; 2) guidance of epilepsy surgery, based on co-localization of evoked potential activity, metabolical and receptor activity related to anatomically and behaviourally derived response[2]; and 3) isolation of specific gyral activation areas related to cognitive performance loss due to sleep deprivation (PET/MRI)[3]. In theory, this fusion technique can be extended to other types of images and spatially derived data, such as evoked potential maps and MRI spectroscopic maps.

This chapter describes the fundamental processes required to apply fusion to brain images, and will illustrate their application related to current research protocols.

Image fusion

Fusion is a process of image superposition, whose primary objective is to facilitate the anatomical interpretation of functional images. It is based on the overlay of different image modalities applied to the same brain regions. Image fusion permits the direct, simultaneous review of various image modalities, each of which highlights different but complementary information. Image fusion provides the functional (PET, SPET) information in an anatomical context provided by the anatomical (MRI or CT) images. Given image data sets that are registered, overlay of congruent planes portray both metabolical activity or blood flow related to the underlying anatomy.

Fusion is accomplished by partitioning the display palette into two distinct colour regimes. The display palette defines the colour or grey-scale mapping representation. For ease of review and because of general familiarity, the anatomical image is usually assigned a grey-scale palette and forms the background or *underlay* image. The functional image is displayed in an *overlay* fashion in a different and visually contrasting palette. This is usually a colour palette which assigns activity levels to colours which are easily interpreted as being ordered. An ordered colour palette assigns the 'cooler' colours to low values and the 'hotter' colours to higher activity values. Automation of the display allows individual image planes to be suppressed or enhanced as required. The colours representing the functional (PET) and anatomical (MRI) images are 'blended' for optimum visual contrast. The contrast of either or both image planes can be adjusted to highlight function or anatomy.

Figs. 1 to 3 show the results of the fusion process for a ^{15}O PET speech discrimination study. In this study paradigm, individual subjects act as their own controls.

In the speech discrimination task, subjects were asked serially to perform various speech perception-dependent tasks, including auditory discrimination, identification and comprehension. During these individual subtasks, specific regions of the brain become activated and are captured in the functional imaging process. Correlation of the regional activity was made with pre-imaging cortical electrical interference and EEG measurements. On the left of Fig. 1 is a transaxial MRI slice at the AC–PC line which serves as the anatomical baseline. The middle image shows the corresponding functional image derived from a registered PET data set.

The right-hand image illustrates the fusion process. Results of the analyses of the fusion images showed that auditory discrimination, identification

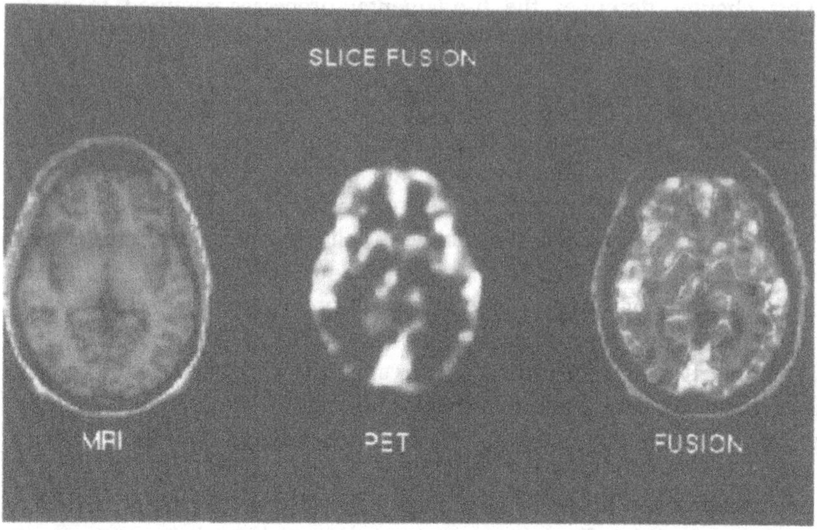

Fig. 1. This Figure shows a set of images from a speech discrimination study. On the left is a transaxial MRI slice at the AC–PC line. Next to it is the corresponding slice from a registered PET data set. The fusion is used to correlate the anatomical regions to the functional metabolical activity level.

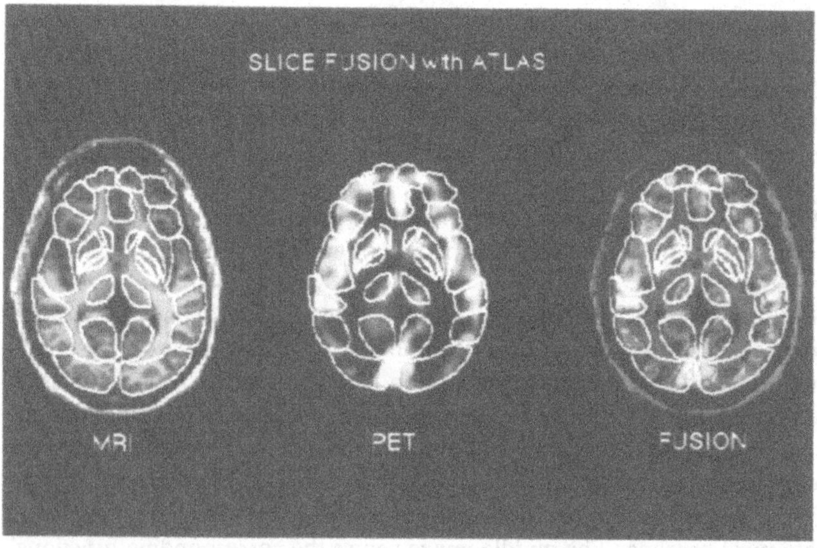

Fig. 2. This Figure shows the same images as in the previous Figure with the MRI-derived atlas fused to each image. This gives a quick visual reference as to the anatomical locations of the regions of high and low metabolical activity.

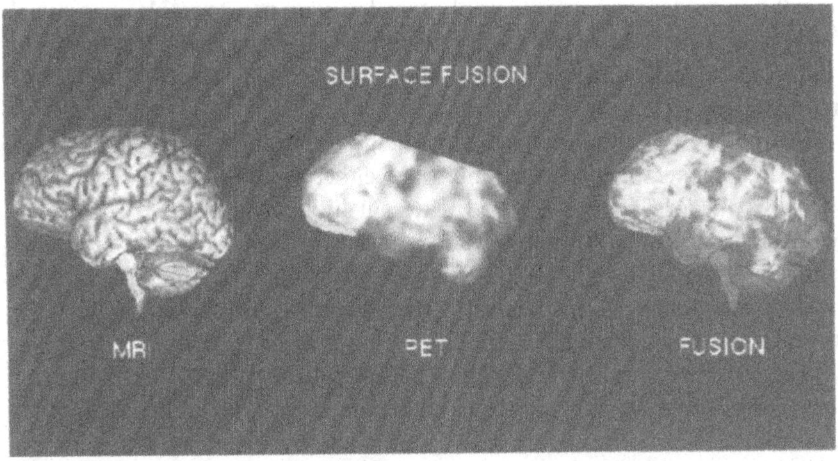

Fig. 3. This Figure shows the left sagittal surface for the same study as in the previous two Figures. With fusion, the regions of high activity are shown to correlate to the mid- and inferior frontal gyri as well as the supra-marginal gyrus.

and comprehension exhibit activity peaks in the superior temporal region. Correlation with pattern of perceptual deficits observed during the electrical interference tests suggests that discrimination and identification operate independently of comprehension (H. Holcomb MD, private communications).

The interpretation process can be enhanced considerably by using an anatomically derived atlas. The atlas for individual subjects is derived by identifying visible edges in the feature-rich anatomical image and fusing this atlas on to the functional image. This is illustrated in Fig. 2 for a mid-plane transaxial slice from the study described above. The atlas provides another derivative plane of information which is helpful in investigating the connectiveness (circuitry) of the behavioural task under investigation.

A similar process is followed for cortical surface images. Fig. 3 shows the results of the fusion process for the cortical surface from the left sagittal view for the study described above. Regions of high activity are located in the middle and inferior frontal gyri with additional activity highlighted in the region corresponding to the supra-marginal gyrus.

Image processing techniques required for functional/anatomical image fusion

Within modality and cross-modality image registration

Without precise registration and an a priori anatomical feature definition, it is difficult correctly to correlate the activity presented in the functional images to specific anatomical regions. The functional image modalities often do not present features which exactly correlate with recognizable anatomical features and hence are not easily interpreted. This is due to the way in which individual brains are 'wired' and to partial volume effects of the imaging technique.

Accurate within and cross-modality image registration form the basis for image fusion. Registration is accomplished either prospectively or retrospectively. In the prospective method, external 'fiducial' reference points are pre-established for both imaging modalities. The term 'fiducial reference point' refers to a pre-established reference point that is identifiable in both imaging modalities. Retrospectively, natural landmarks are used in either a direct or an iterated 'fitting' procedure.

In general, 'rigid body' registration involves three steps: 1) extraction of common features (natural or fiducial) in the target and object image; 2) determination of the transformation parameters by matching the common features in the target and object images; and 3) mathematical transformation and digital remapping of the images.

The techniques (which assume that the brain is a 'rigid body') which are currently used and for which validation has been accomplished include: 1) matching with external landmarks[4,5]; 2) matching surfaces by minimizing 'distances'[6]; 3) matching spatial moments (centroids, principal axes)[7,8]; and 4) correlation techniques[9–11]. Registration, then, is implemented by determining from three to six coordinate parameters (three translations, three rotations), and using these parameters to calculate the transformed coordinates of the base image. The accuracy of registration of these various techniques are of the order 0.5–1.5 mm at the centre of the brain. Accuracies from 1 to 4 mm at the cortical surface have been demonstrated.

Image warping

Since there is, in general, significant spatial variation of the anatomical features in the human brain[12], the matching of individual subjects and the averaging process for group subjects often require a process of *image warping*. Warping is a piecewise process which defines the spatial transformation required to match digital images from different subjects or to match a specific subject to a single reference brain or to a generalized atlas. Warping redefines the spatial relationship between a specific identifiable set of common reference landmarks in each image. A common reference for group data can be a stylized atlas (such as that produced by Talairach[13]), or a common brain projection (such as made by averaging MRI images from a number of subjects). Image warping is sometimes called 'rubber-sheeting' because of the analogy of variable stretching, which can be conceived by subjecting a rubber sheet to variable local elevation perturbations.

Warping techniques were developed by Smythe[14] at Industrial Light and Magic to generate special visual effects, such as the smooth series of object

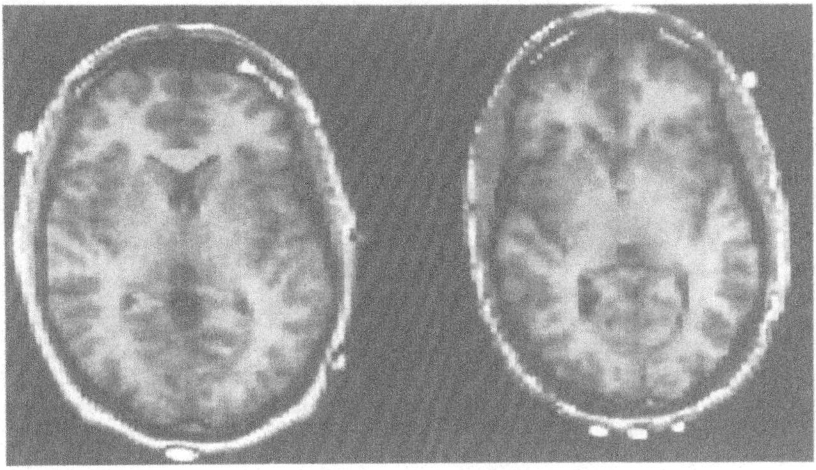

Fig. 4. Two slices are shown from two different subjects. The slices were acquired at the AC–PC plane for each subject.

transforms from goat, to ostrich, to turtle, to tiger, to woman. For the brain, we transform recognizable objects, such as gyri, from their original shape into a standard composited, gyral shape. The process for image warping generally proceeds by first defining an image distortion model. The distortion model defines the transformation between the landmarks in the target and object image data set. The distortion model is defined by the series of reference points or fiducials which are determined discretely in each image.

In the warping technique, the input and output image (source and destination images) are partitioned into a mesh of patches. Each patch defines a specific contiguous region of the image in which a uniform mapping function is applied. This is done by selecting a discrete set of recognizable landmarks which are visible in both images. The mapping function is defined strictly only for these points. The mapping function transforms each patch in the input image on to its corresponding region in the output image. Since a rectangular topology is imposed on the mesh points, any bivariate function may be fitted to the data, providing that there is no folding or discontinuity. Figs. 4 to 6 illustrate the warping process.

The development of image data sets enabled by the registration/fusion process

Image subtraction paradigms

Recent advances in functional imaging technology have led to techniques for determining behaviourally based activity using a repeated behavioural task paradigm[15]. Task-related activation is determined by the subtraction of

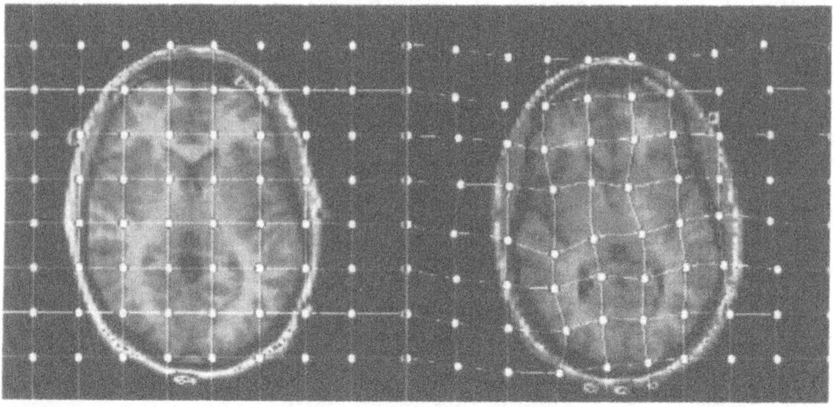

Fig. 5. A grid is superimposed on each slice. The user then places the points on corresponding anatomical features. A fit is calculated and the image is warped accordingly.

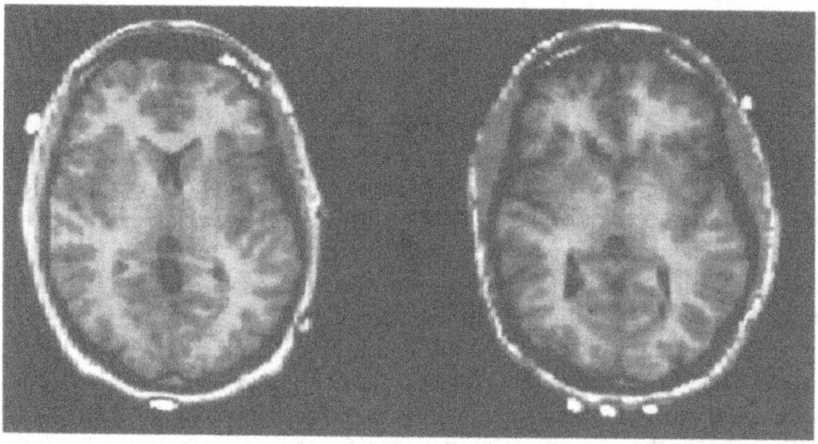

Fig. 6. The right slice has been warped to spatially match the left image. A similar fit can be used to warp registered functional images, such as PET or SPECT.

a control (baseline) task from various levels or types of activated tasks. In these paradigms the subject is his/her own control. Areas of significant difference are determined by subjecting the subtraction images (specific behavioural task – registered baseline task) to a statistical analysis based on the frequency of clusters of graded activation. The significance of activity differences is based on the statistical probability of finding clusters above the level of those occurring at random.

Subtraction studies are done on single subjects in a repeated behavioural paradigm or in experiments that are repeated on groups of subjects where the subtracted images are transformed into a common stereotactic space and averaged. Based on a subtraction paradigm, Roland[16] computed that the probability of finding activation cluster changes above 15% in statistically spatially independent pixels is less than 5% in noise-only images.

Particularly for functional imaging modalities, the smallest imaging element, the voxel, is generally smaller than the spatial resolution of the scanner. This means that neighbouring voxels are correlated. This effect can be investigated by analysing the auto-correlation in primarily noise-dominated images. The underlying statistical hypothesis of functional images, particularly functional subtraction images, is that there is statistically significant change in the activation fields.

The fusion process, overlaying the functional image on to the anatomical image substrate, is particularly useful for the interpretation of images in these repeat behavioural task paradigms since the images are self-registered. Clusters of high activity change are indicative of the involvement of different regions in an activated state task. While these clusters do not usually take the form of anatomically identified features, the superposition of identified anatomical features aids in anatomical association. Anatomical association is accomplished by stereotactic localization or by fusion to a recognizable anatomical substrate.

Fig. 7 illustrates the use of the subtraction paradigm in an experiment where the effect of noise on word identification is investigated. The baseline task is produced by simple repetitive button pressing. In the activated state, a correct identification of a word is also signified by pressing a button. The effect of button pressing is eliminated in the subtraction image.

Proper interpretation of the subtraction images is enhanced significantly by registering the total image data set to an anatomical base image such as derived from MRI. The use of subtraction imaging paradigms requires that the individual images from each task variant or time point be carefully registered since subtraction is a noise enhancer.

Anatomical to functional image fusion can provide the necessary spatial–interpretive link between existing generalized functional information representation and specific pattern localization based on the anatomical features of individual subjects. Techniques have been developed to functionally dissect behavioural tasks by mapping activation profile differences using 3D functional/anatomical fusion in a repeated PET imaging paradigm[3]. These techniques provide information on activation patterns related to gyral and sulcal landmarks, internal landmarks or common stereotactic spatial reference systems.

Group averaging

Fox and Mintun[17] and Fox et al[18] developed the technique of intersubject averaging to improve the signal-to-noise ratio of PET subtraction images.

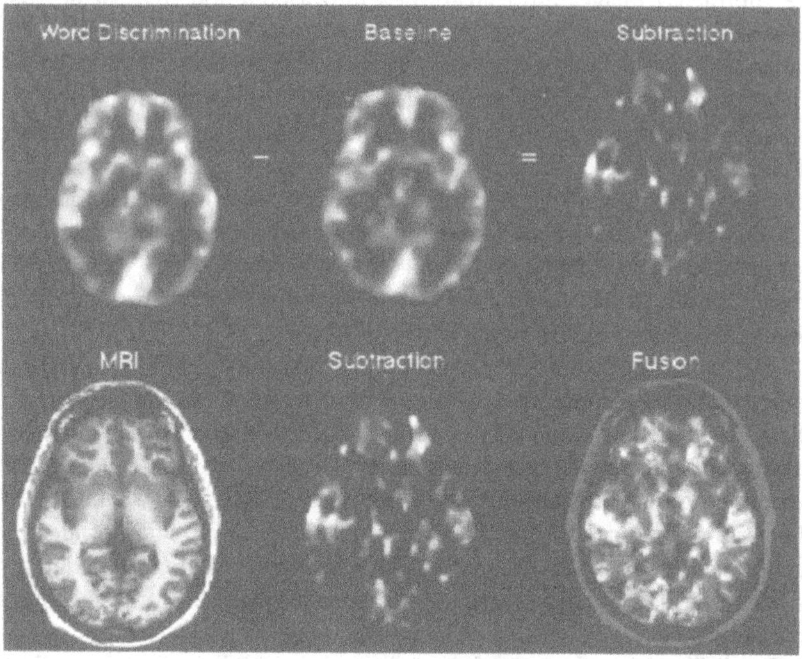

Fig. 7. Subtraction is used to show the metabolical pattern of the target task (speech discrimination) by removing the effects of the baseline task (button pressing). The resultant subtraction image is difficult to interpret anatomically. With fusion, the regions of high activity are shown to be in the superior temporal and superior frontal gyri.

Group averaging

Fox and Mintun[17] and Fox et al[18] developed the technique of intersubject averaging to improve the signal-to-noise ratio of PET subtraction images. This technique was specifically developed to map higher order, non-primary activation areas with highly focal, low activity level differences. The technique is based on the hypothesis that, in the averaging process, random background noise cancels itself out while consistent focal activity increases with the number of images.

Combining individual subject images into a single group pattern is an important tool in current experiment strategies. Fig. 8 illustrates the process of forming group images from similar tasks performed by a number of different individuals. Group registration is performed by warping the individual subject planar images to a common reference image. Group images of average activity for both direct and subtraction algorithms allow the development of statistical parameter maps. Absolute and subtracted activity levels can be displayed by using the statistical information from repeated experi-

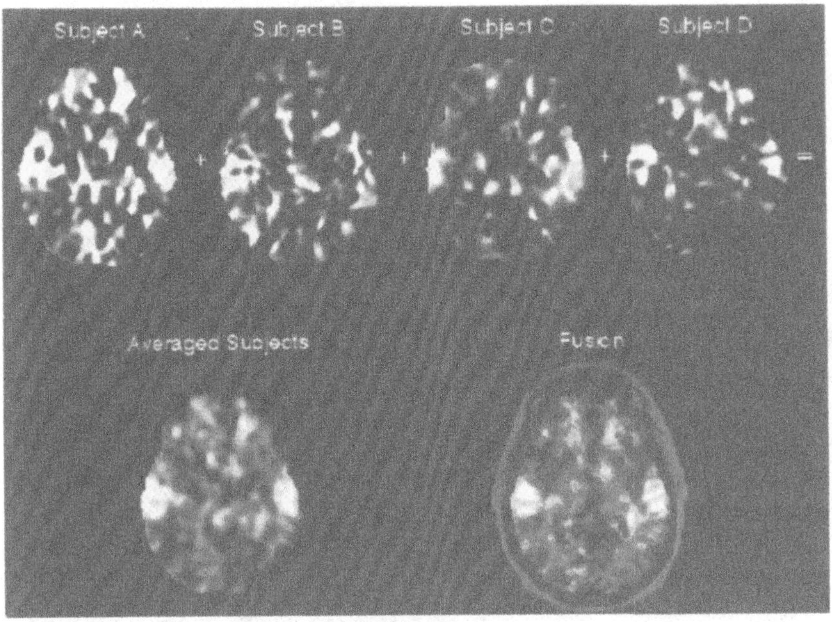

Fig. 8. Slices from different normal subjects performing the same task are shown. The PET data set from each subject were registered to their own MRI. Then a slice was obtained from the AC–PC line of each. After warping the slices of each subject to one base subject using the MRI slice as a template, the average of the PET slices for all four subjects can be calculated. The resultant image can be fused to the MRI from the base subject.

ments or groups to generate *t*-maps, *z*-score maps, χ^2-maps, etc. These statistical maps generally consider that the computed voxels are independent, even though near voxels are generally correlated owing to the acquisition process.

Using the activity values of the total volume (or the total grey matter volume), a *z*-score transformation of the data can be used to normalize subject to subject. The *z*-score normalizes the activity data according to the relationship:

$$z = \frac{x - \bar{x}}{\sigma}$$

where x = activity value in a specific region of interest
$\bar{x}$ = mean activity of the slice or volume
σ = standard deviation of the slice or volume

z-scoring transforms the mean to a 0 reference and puts the data in units of standard deviation. Fig. 9 shows the overlay of the *z*-score mapping on

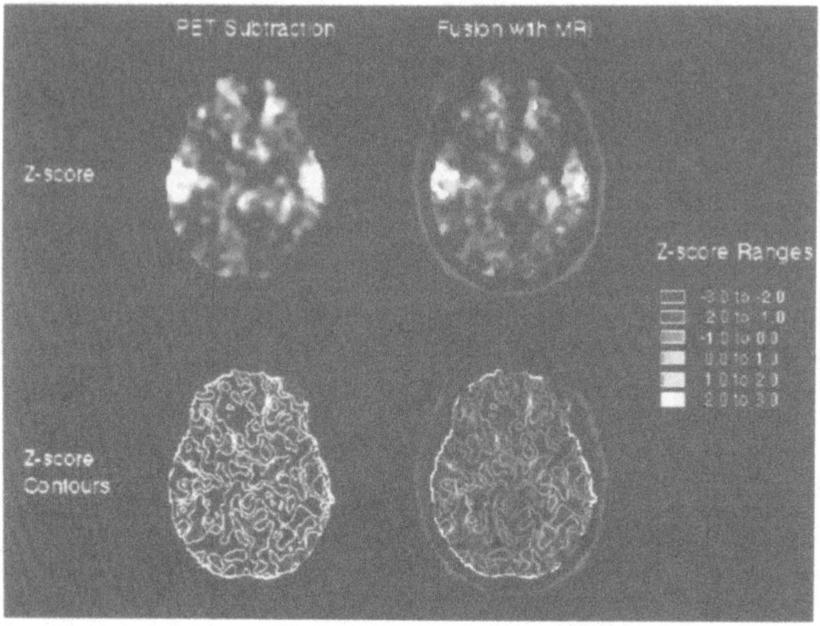

Fig. 9. Shown above is the z-score mapping for a subtraction image. The z-score mapping simplifies the determination of regions of high and low activity. Fusion with the MRI allows for easy visualization of the regions of interest, which, in this case, is the superior temporal gyri.

to mid-plane transaxial images shown previously. By combining the z-score with cluster statistics[17,18,21,22], the statistical significance of these activity clusters can be determined.

In group averaging the process of image warping based on anatomically registered images is used to develop a single composite image of the group. The fusion of co-registered slices and surfaces significantly enhances the interpretation of the images and the correlation of activation foci and clusters related to task-dependent brain activity.

Individual neuroanatomical variability can compromise the use of group averaging for enhancing activation signal to noise. Additionally, the subject-to-subject variability of brain shape gyral patterns, and subgyral connectivity, may not be covered by a scaling transformation to an anatomical standard mapping. Steinmetz[12] reports that the scatter of functional sites may be of the order of several centimetres. Proportional spatial transforms do not adjust internal brain configurations separately. Acting as an overall confounder is the fact that individual cognitive strategies are variable. These factors can lead to underestimation of the amount of association involved in cognitive studies using group averaging. Galaburda[19] has shown that the cytoarchitectronic boundaries can exhibit significant variability with respect to the structural landmarks of the brain. To this variability must be factored in considerations that: 1) individual cognitive strategy is variable; and 2) the degree of functional lateralization is variable.

Subject-specific and subject-averaged anatomical atlases

A benefit of the general processes involved in providing fusion of functional/anatomical information is the capability to develop subject-specific and subject-averaged anatomical atlas overlays. Based on the development of high resolution, isotropic anatomical data sets, it has become feasible to develop surface–volumetric depictions of the brain. Surface images clearly show identifiable sulcal landmarks which can serve as a basis for a cortical surface atlas.

The development of subject-specific atlases provides a technique for automated region of interest sampling since the anatomically derived regions of interest match all successive registered image data sets. For example, the surface-derived atlas for a subject under a repeated imaging paradigm for evaluating the effect of sleep deprivation on cognitive performance is shown in Fig. 10. The atlas allows anatomical interpretation of the cortical sagittal surface pattern related to specific behavioural tasks. The pattern shows a generalized decrease in metabolical activity for increased sleep deprivation.

Fig. 11 is an example of a cortical surface image constructed using MRI. Using the sulci as a boundary demarcation a gyral atlas can be developed easily as shown to the right. The cortical surface can also be 'peeled' to reveal the underlying convolutions of individual gyri as shown in Fig. 12. Similar atlases can be developed for subcortical structures.

Atlases can be used in automatic regions of interest sampling by projection of the digitally obtained regions from the anatomical substrate on to the functional images. This greatly reduces the time involved in developing anatomically based interpretation of subtraction paradigms and in the development of statistical pattern vectors.

Applications of image fusion

There are three major application types which require or benefit from functional/anatomical image registration and fusion techniques: 1) functional dissection; 2) activation task profiles; and 3) statistical activity clustering.

Functional dissection

Functional dissection is a term that defines the specification of region of interest (ROI) activation based on the projection of functional data on to a registered and identified anatomical substrate (specific nuclei, gyri, sulcal position, etc.).

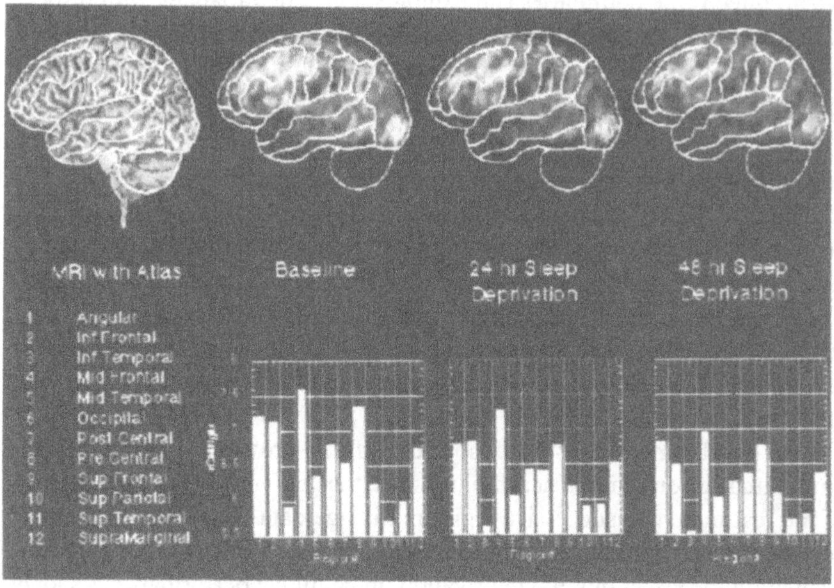

Fig. 10. Fusion of the atlas to the anatomical and functional images allows the precise location of regions of interest that can be used for repeated imaging paradigms. In this sleep deprivation study, the atlas derived from the MRI surface is used to sample on the baseline and two sleep deprivation time points. The graphs show that a generalized decrease in metabolical activity correlates to increased sleep deprivation.

The major objective of functional dissection is to map the activation fields related to specific tasks on the cytoarchitecture of the brain, and to provide a standard stereotactic reference frame for the centroid and extent of specific activity fields.

One of the benefits of relating functional activation to anatomical landmarks is to allow individual experiment comparisons with the large ad hoc body of brain mapping[4] information related to the brain's cytoarchitecture which currently exists and which is in the process of being incorporated into comprehensive databases.

Activation task profiles (ROI activation pattern vectors)

Activation task profiles (ATPs) are measured ROI activity values defined relative to independently identified anatomical features. ATPs are constructed by organizing ROI values from selected brain areas into activity vectors or 'profiles'. These profiles represent an arbitrary, but defined, arrangement of anatomical features. ATPs can be indicative of the associ-

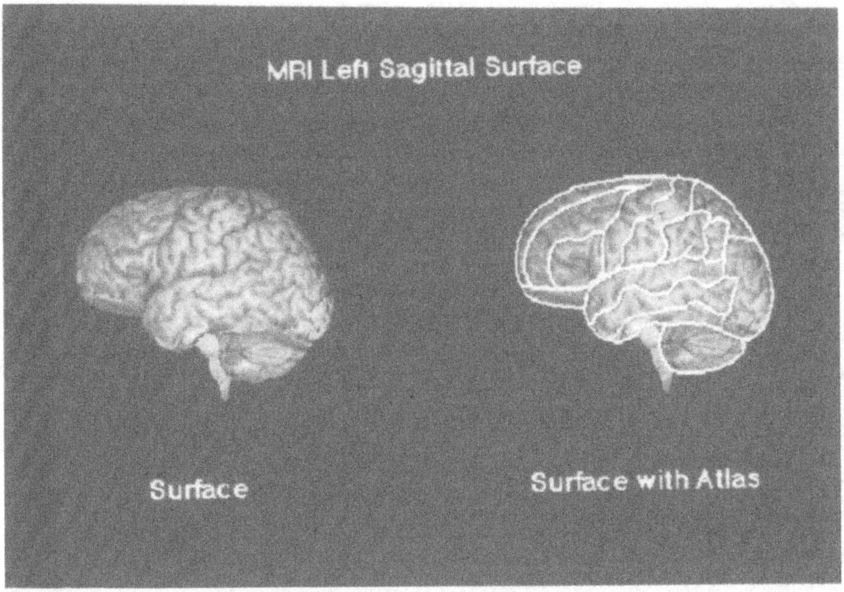

Fig. 11. Example of a cortical surface image constructed using MRI volume data set. Using the sulci as a boundary demarcation, a gyral atlas can be easily developed as shown to the right.

ation between anatomically determined regions and behavioural task activation, and can contribute important information relating to the connectivity of the brain. They are particularly useful for interpreting subtraction-based comparisons of tasks derived from repeated tests using a subject as his own control.

For example, Kippenhan et al[20] used a pattern vector approach to classify Alzheimer (AD) versus normal patients based on FDG–PET images. They input the regional metabolical patterns into a neural network pattern classifier to separate normal and abnormal (AD) patients. In a diagnostic setting the profiles represent n-dimensional discrimination surfaces which define the 'pattern-space' direction of increasing severity of disease (n refers to the number of regions in the profile). Kippenhan and co-workers also concluded from this effort that it is possible to successfully combine normalized data from a different database.

The activation task profile methodology requires anatomical/functional fusion since this approach inherently suffers from spatial dilution effects. If the a priori ROI are large relative to the area activated during the specific task, the relative difference between the task-specific and background areas

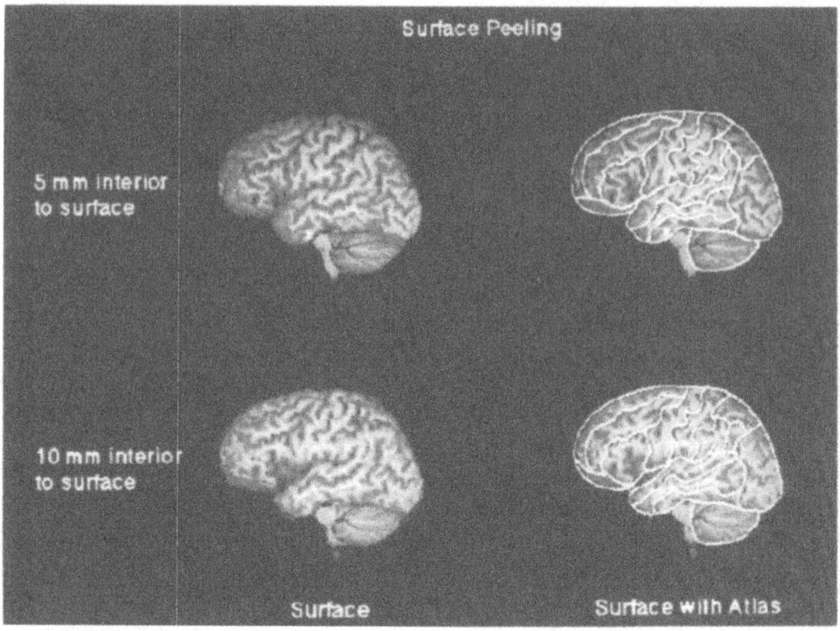

Fig. 12. Images can be made interior to the surface of the brain. Here, images are created 5 and 10 mm interior to the surface. Using this method, the whole volume of a gyrus can be visualized.

will be reduced. This compromises the capability of using the activation pattern vector approach based solely on easily recognized features such as the gyri.

Activity localization based on clustering statistics

Statistical clustering techniques and parameter maps were introduced by Friston et al[21] to interpret subtraction paradigm images. Registered data sets allow the formation of *z*-score or *t*-statistic images. Based on threshold values of the statistic, a clustering technique is used to identify those regions with specified statistical significance. These techniques are also required in the statistical approaches of Worsley[22] (Montreal) and the more recently developed statistical approach which combines activity level with cluster size developed by Poline and Mazoyer[23] in France.

Future developments of fusion techniques

The ever-increasing availability of image computing power at rapidly lowering cost is fostering the ability to use more complex imaging strategies for the interpretation of activation of the brain. While primarily used in research settings, the capability to register and compare anatomical and functional information will steadily find increasing use in clinical settings.

The variability of the spatial positions of function on individual brains increases the value of the stereotactic projection of functional activity and further supports the use of independently determined anatomical identification aided by the fusion process. Accurate temporal registration and fusion could aid significantly in defining subtle recurrent disease and serve to identify the functional aspects of atrophy and gradual dementing illness.

Functional analysis of the human brain based on cerebral blood flow or cerebral metabolism, derived primarily from PET, SPET and functional MRI images, has been shown to contribute valuable and otherwise unobtainable information related to cognitive studies and functional connectivity. Posner[1] laid the basis for the use of anatomically interpreted functional imaging related to cognitive/behavioural studies of the brain by positing that: 1) a set of distributed brain areas must be orchestrated in the performance of even simple tasks; and 2) even though each task is not localized to a specific single area, the operations which comprise the task are strictly localized.

Critical to understanding the functioning and connectivity of the brain is the ability to measure both the brain areas which are activated during a particular behavioural or cognitive task, and the time course of information exchange among these brain areas. The study of the functioning and connectivity of the brain relies on the ability to define the relationship between anatomy, function and timing, leading to the use of combined MRI, PET, SPET and functional MRI imaging.

Carefully constructed cognitive experiments using a baseline *control state* subtracted from an activated *task state* have recently made it possible to identify brain functional areas (activity fields) involved in the mental operations unique to each task state.

In addition to regional glucose metabolism and blood flow (PET and SPET) techniques, the rapidly developing techniques of functional MRI[2] (fMRI) will play an increasingly important role as neurophysiological imaging probes.

Acknowledgement

The authors would like to thank Dr Henry Holcomb of the Maryland Psychiatric Institute for providing the PET and MRI data for use in this effort.

References

(1) Posner MI, Petersen SE, Fox PT, Raichle ME. Localization of cognitive operations in the human brain. *Science* 1988; 240: 1627–31.

(2) Belliveau JW, Kennedy DN, McKinstry RC et al. Functional mapping of the

human visual cortex by magnetic resonance imaging. *Science* 1991; 254: 716–19.
(3) Loats H. *Cortical surface metabolic mapping.* Proceedings of Third International Peace Through Mind/Brain Science. 1990; Hammamatsu, Japan.
(4) Loats H. CT and SPECT image registration and fusion for spatial localization of metastatic processes using radiolabeled monoclonals. *J Nucl Med* 1993; 000: 562–6.
(5) Toga AW, ed. *Three-dimensional neuroimaging.* Raven Press; 1990.
(6) Pelizzari CA, Chen GTY, Spelbring DR, Weichselbaum RR, Chen CT. Accurate three-dimensional registration of CT PET, and/or MR images of the brain. *J Comp Ass Tomog* 1989; 13: 20–6.
(7) Rusinek H, Tsui W, Levy AV, Noz ME, deLeon MJ. Principal axes and surface fitting methods for three-dimensional image registration. *J Nucl Med* 1993; 34(11): 2019–24.
(8) a. Levy AV, Brodie JD, Russell JAG, Volkow ND, Laska E, Wolf AP. The metabolic centroid method for PET brain image analysis. *J Cereb Blood Flow Metab* 1989; 9: 388–97.
b. Levy AV, Laska E, Brodie JD, Volkow ND, Wolf AP. The spectral signature method for the analysis of PET brain images. *J Cereb Blood Flow Metab* 1991; 11: A103–13.
c. Levy AV, Volkow ND, Brodie JD, Bertollo DN, Wolf AP. The spectral analysis of brain glucose metabolism. *Proceedings of the 12th Annual International Conference of the IEEE Engineering in Medicine and Biology* 1990; 12(3): 1299–301.
(9) Hoh CK (UCLA Medical Center) Dohbohm, Harris G, Choi Y, Hawkins R, Phelps M, Maddahi J. Automated iterative three-dimensional registration of position tomography images. *J Nucl Med* 1993; 34: 2009–18.
(10) Woods RP (UCLA School of Medicine), Simon CR, Mazziotta JC. Rapid automated algorithm for aligning and reslicing PET images. *J Comp Ass Tomog* 1992; 16(4): 620–33.
(11) Hibbard LS, Hawkins RA. Objective image alignment for three-dimensional reconstruction of digital autoradiograms. *J Neurosci Methods* 1988; 26: 528.
(12) Steinmetz H, Seitz RJ. Functional anatomy of language processing: neuroimaging and the problem of individual variability. *Neuropsychology* 1991; 29(12): 1149–61.
(13) Talairach J, Tournoux P. *Co-planar stereotaxic atlas of the human brain 3-D dimensional proportional system: an approach to cerebral imaging.* New York: Thième Medical Publishers, Inc.; 1988.
(14) Symthe DB. A two-pass mesh warping algorithm for object transformation and image interpolation. *ILM Technical Memo 1030*, Computer Graphics Department, Lucasfilm Ltd; 1990.
(15) Raichle M. Visualizing the mind. *Sci Am* 1994; Apr: 58–64.
(16) Roland PE. *Brain activation.* Wiley-Liss; 1993.
(17) Fox PL, Mintun MA. Noninvasive functional brain mapping by change-distribution analysis of averaged PET images of $H_2{}^{15}O$ tissue activity. *Clin Sci* 1989; 30(2).
(18) Fox PL, Mintun MA, Reiman EM, Raichle ME. Enhanced detection of focal

brain responses using intersubject averaging and change-distribution analysis of subtracted PET images. *J Cereb Blood Flow Metab* 1988; 8: 642–53.

(19) Galaburda A, Sanides F. Cytoarchitectonic organization of the human auditory cortex. *J Comp Neurol* 1980; 190: 597–610.

(20) Kippenhan JS, Barker W, Pascal S, Nagel J, Duara R. Evaluation of a neural-network classifier for PET scans of normal and Alzheimer's disease subjects. *J Nucl Med* 1992; 33(8): 000–00.

(21) Friston KJ, Frith CD, Liddle PF, Frackowiak RSF. Comparing functional (PET) images: the assessment of significant change. *J Cereb Blood Flow Metab* 1991; 11: 690–9.

(22) Worsley KJ, Evans AC, Marrett S, Neelin P. A three dimensional statistical analysis for CBF activation studies in human brain. *J Cereb Blood Flow Metab* 1992; 12: 900–18.

(23) Poline JP, Mazoyer B. Analysis of individual positron emission tomography activation maps by detection of high signal–noise ratio pixel clusters. *J Cereb Blood Flow Metab* 1993; 13(3): 245–437.

Development of SPET as a tool for neuropsychopharmacological research

J P SEIBYL

Introduction

Single photon emission computed tomography (SPET) imaging has been available for over 30 years dating back to pioneering work by Kuhl who applied backprojection algorithms to reconstruct tomographic images of objects scanned at different angles[1]. Despite these early efforts, tomographic brain imaging with SPET was eclipsed by transmission tomographic techniques and by interest in development of positron emission tomography (PET). It is only within the past decade, following the availability of new radiotracers for imaging brain perfusion and receptor distribution, that brain SPET has undergone revitalization as both a clinical and research tool[2].

The utility of SPET for studying aspects of brain function is underscored by the development of promising new methods for neuropsychopharmacological investigations to the study of neuropsychiatric disease and the mechanisms of psychotropic drug action.

SPET cerebral blood flow vs receptor studies

SPET brain scans may be divided into examinations of cerebral flow or brain receptor studies. These studies provide different and often complementary information about brain function. Both [^{99m}Tc]- and [^{123}I]-labelled SPET tracers are used to image brain perfusion based on the premise that in most circumstances blood flow is tightly coupled to cellular metabolism and thus provides an indirect measure of neuronal metabolic rate[3]. Blood flow within any brain region is determined by multiple cellular events involving both glia and neurones, and includes the excitatory and inhibitory influences of nerve cells located within the region of interest as well as metabolism within presynaptic terminals originating from distant

All correspondence to: Professor J P Seibyl, Departments of Diagnostic Radiology and Psychiatry, Yale University School of Medicine, TE-2, 333 Cedar Street, New Haven, CT 06520, USA.

Cambridge Medical Reviews: Neurobiology and Psychiatry Volume 3

neurones projectioning to the area. These events are integrated over the time of incorporation of radiotracer into brain.

Properties of radiotracer uptake and washout from brain are important to interpretation of the study. Agents like [^{99m}Tc]HM-PAO are taken up into cells within minutes of injection and exhibit negligible washout from cells. Images represent brain perfusion over the short interval of incorporation into cells, regardless of when the actual SPET scan is obtained. [^{123}I]iodoamphetamine is rapidly distributed to brain but undergoes washout and redistribution, thus the SPET images represent events occurring over a longer time integral and are sensitive to the time of scan acquisition. Both tracers capture dynamic patterns of brain blood flow and are affected potentially by sensory stimulation, motor activation, mood and cognitive state of the subject[4].

In distinction to blood flow, SPET receptor studies offer greater discrimination of specific neuronal populations based on the heterogenous brain distribution of these cells and their associated receptor sites. Receptors are the target of both neurotransmitter substances and most psychotropic drugs; hence, neuroreceptor SPET may be considered a measure of in vivo neurochemistry and is well suited for neuropharmacological research. SPET receptor studies are potentially less sensitive to such factors as the subject's cognitive set or level of sensory activation. This chapter will consider only SPET receptor studies.

SPET and PET neuroreceptor studies

SPET receptor studies have been considered subordinate to positron emission tomography (PET) receptor examinations with regard to number of available radioligands and algorithms for quantitating regional brain receptor density (B_{max}). Issues of lower photon flux, poorer resolution and the requirement of accurate correction schemes for scattered and attenuated photons frustrate acquisiton of quantitative brain SPET data. Despite this, the lower cost, ready availability of SPET imaging systems and lack of requirement for on-site isotope production makes the wider application of clinically useful SPET studies feasible[2]. A subtle advantage of SPET over PET lies in the use of longer-lived isotopes which offer greater flexibility in study design including the evaluation of brain activity up to 24 h post-tracer administration and protocols involving radiotracer administration as a continuous infusion over several hours described below.

Role of neuroreceptor SPET in neuropsychopharmacology

SPET neuroreceptor studies provide information about the pharmacokinetics, brain uptake and biodistribution of radioligands selective for brain receptor targets. Neuronal receptors are the targets for both endogenous neurotransmitter and many psychotropic drugs. Hence, SPET can be used to evaluate the receptor occupancy of psychotropic drugs which compete with radiotracer for receptor binding. These assessments may be performed by comparison of SPET scans obtained during unmedicated baseline and drug treatment conditions[5] or during the infusion of the test drug during dynamic, multiple SPET acquisitions[6]. In addition, SPET can provide estimates of the distribution and number of receptor sites that are subject to disturbance in neuropsychiatric disease or as a consequence of drug treatment. SPET may detect *increased* receptor density in cases of receptor upregulation such as occurring during treatment with agents that antagonize receptor function or *decreases* in receptor binding occurring with neuronal loss or downregulation of receptors on intact neurones. Major advantages of SPET over in vitro evaluations of receptor binding include information about the in vivo behaviour of radiotracer or test drugs which includes consideration of such factors as penetrance of blood–brain barrier, peripheral metabolism and body clearance[7].

General principles and algorithms for studying brain receptors with SPET

SPET outcome measures

Absolute quantitation of the SPET signal is not required for estimation of in vivo drug receptor binding when the measure is expressed as the percentage of occupied binding sites. However, SPET evaluation of receptor distribution and number requires an outcome measure linearly proportional to the density of receptors (B_{max}) within brain. Absolute SPET measures of receptor density have been elusive leading most investigators to adopt semiquantitative analytic methods in most clinical and pre-clinical SPET neuroreceptor applications. None the less, recent work demonstrates the feasibility of truly quantitative algorithms with SPET[8,9].

Standard approaches to SPET data analysis

The ratio of the concentration of detected counts (expressed as counts/pixel/min) in receptor-rich brain regions to a reference area devoid of receptors or whole brain is the most commonly utilized SPET outcome measure. Ratio measurements are easy to calculate and correct for day-to-day differences in camera sensitivity, administered dose of radiotracer, physical decay and brain uptake between test subjects. However, ratio measurements are sensitive to time of SPET sampling due to variability in the rate of tracer washout from different brain regions. Specifically, the target:reference region ratio of counts increases with time as brain regions with negligible receptor densities exhibit faster tracer washout than receptor-rich regions (Fig. 1). The clearance of tracer from the circulating blood pool dictates the washout rate from regions with negligible receptor numbers. Thus, the

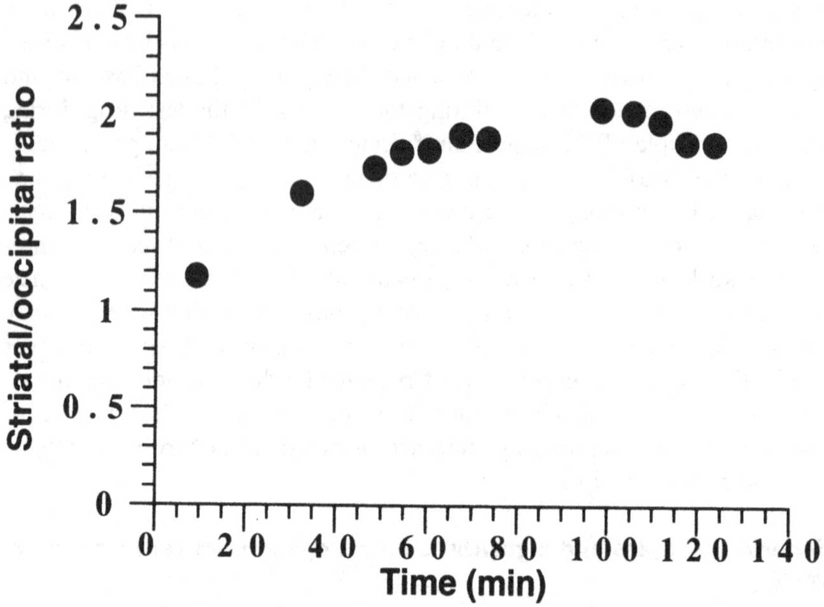

Fig. 1. Ratio of activity in striatum to occipital cortex in human subject receiving bolus injection of [^{123}I]IBZM. The ratio increases over the course of the examination because the rate of radiotracer washout is faster from the receptor-poor occipital cortex than from the receptor-rich striatum.

major limitation of ratio methods lies in the non-linearity of this measure to B_{max} and dependence on metabolism and peripheral clearance which may be highly variable between test subjects.

A second SPET outcome measure suggested by limitations of ratio methods entails analysis of regional brain time–activity data. Three common measures obtained from the radioactive decay-corrected curves are the time to peak counts, amplitude of the peak and rate of count washout expressed as percentage washout per hour or the half-life of an exponential curve fit to the post-peak data[10]. Brain areas rich in receptors demonstrate prolonged time to peak uptake, higher peak counts and delayed washout compared with receptor-poor regions (Fig. 2). Regional brain time–activity washout analyses suffer from high between-subject variability caused by differences in the rate of clearance of radiotracer from plasma.

The estimate of washout rate from brain is also dependent on the relative grey:white matter composition within the region of interest (ROI) (Fig. 3). Since white matter is devoid of receptors, the time to peak uptake and washout are rapid and dependent upon the peripheral levels of free parent tracer. Large regions of interest that include a significant proportion of either white matter or brain regions with low receptor numbers will peak earlier at lower

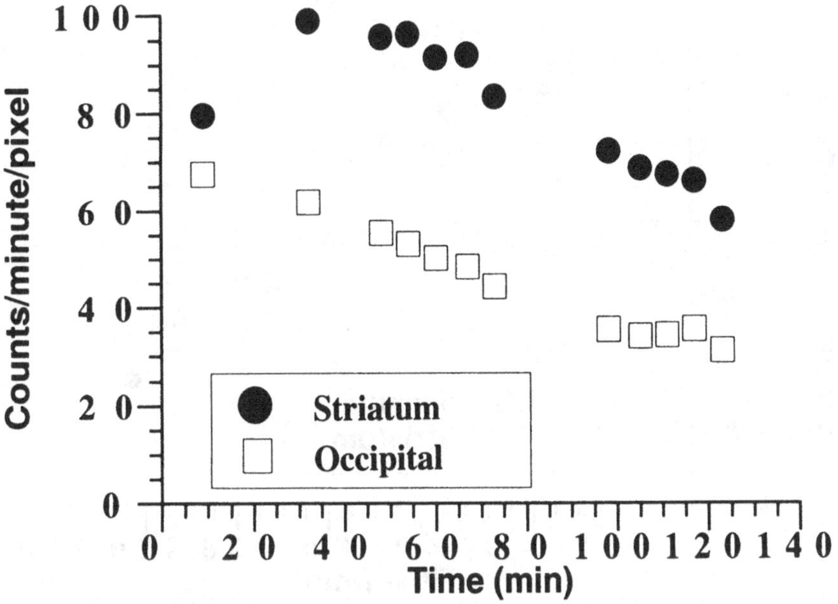

Fig. 2. Regional brain SPET time–activity data in a healthy subject receiving a bolus injection of [^{123}I]IBZM. Regions rich in receptors (striatum) achieve peak uptake later and washout at a slower rate than receptor-poor areas (occipital).

density of counts and washout faster than small regions of interest placed within receptor-rich grey matter.

Body temperature also affects regional brain activity time to peak and washout rates in animal studies utilizing general anaesthesia[7]. Lower body temperatures are associated with slower washout of tracer from brain, presumably due to decreased peripheral metabolism or slower renal clearance. Temperature effects are less critical in human SPET examinations.

In summary, analyses of regional brain time–activity data for estimating regional brain receptor concentration is compromised by the fact that factors unrelated to B_{max} like peripheral clearance, the proportion of grey and white matter within a ROI and the animal's body temperature affects the time to peak regional brain uptake and rate of tracer washout (Table 1).

SPET quantitation of drug receptor binding

Two strategies using neuroreceptor SPET have been successfully applied to the in vivo calculation of receptor occupancy by psychotropic drugs. Neither approach requires absolute quantitation of radioactivity. In the first, subjects receive unmedicated baseline SPET examinations followed by repeated study after a period of treatment with the pharmacological agent. Reductions in specific uptake (i.e. activity associated with binding at the

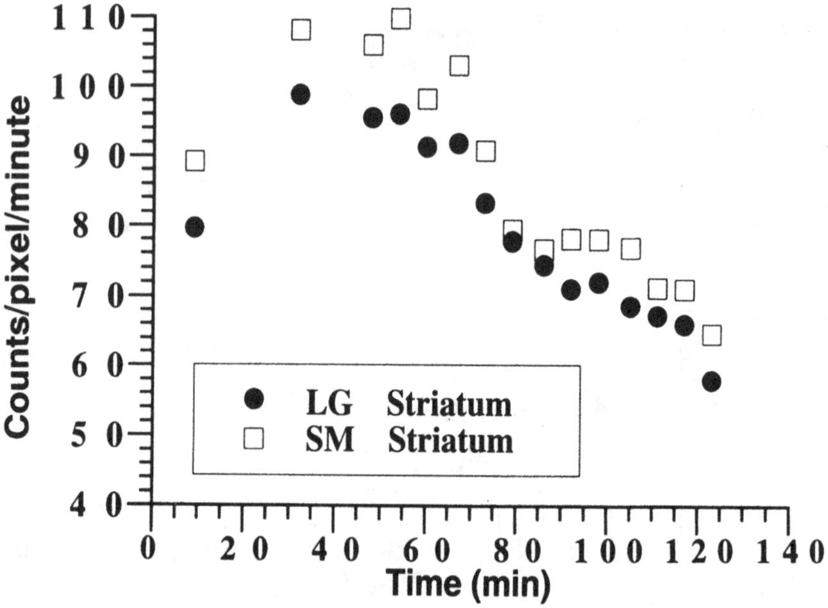

Fig. 3. Time–activity data from dynamic SPET study following the bolus injection of [^{123}I]IBZM in healthy human subject. Activity in the striatum is sampled with a large (lg striatum) and small (sm striatum) region of interest (ROI). The larger ROI produces smoother time–activity data but earlier time to peak uptake and overall lower density of counts (counts/pixel/min) as more receptor-poor areas are included in the sampled region.

Table 1. *Factors affecting rates of regional brain radiotracer washout*

1. Receptor density (B_{max}) and affinity ($1/K_d$) of tracer for the binding site
2. Physiochemical properties of the radioligand (e.g. lipophilicity)
3. Region of interest size and placement
4. Clearance of free parent tracer from the vascular pool
   - Body temperature
   - Metabolism
   - Renal excretion (affected by state of hydration, renal function)
   - Plasma protein binding

target receptor) are expressed as a percentage of the baseline measurement. PET examinations of drug occupancy use this approach[11,12] owing to the short half-life of PET isotopes. The method requires accurate registration of the baseline and drug treatment images for reliable and reproducible brain ROI placement.

A second method for determining psychotropic drug receptor occupancy involves infusion of the test drug during dynamic SPET imaging. Drugs which compete with the radioligand for receptor binding significantly increase the washout rate of radiotracer from receptor-rich brain regions. The displacing drug produces a rapid reduction of brain activity until a plateau is achieved. Areas with low density or negligible receptor numbers are unaffected by the displacing agent.

Radioligands occupy approximately 0.01–0.1% of total receptors with random distribution among the target sites. Thus, for a 'chaser' drug to produce detectable washout of activity the drug must occupy significant numbers of receptors. Analysis of time–activity data of activity associated with specific binding to the receptor allows calculation of the percentage receptor occupancy of the displacing agent according to the following formula:

$$\text{Percentage receptor occupancy by displacing drug} = 100 - \left(\frac{\text{Specific uptake after drug}}{\text{Specific uptake baseline}} \times 100 \right) \quad (1)$$

Serial administrations of the displacing drug produces additional washout until all activity representing specific receptor binding has been displaced (Fig. 4). For studies where multiple serial injections of displacing drug are administered within a scanning session, the logit transformed percentage specific binding (equal to $\ln [P/100-P]$, where P is the percentage displacement) plotted against the cumulative injected dose of displacing drug permits calculation of the displacing drug's in vivo potency, ED_{50}; i.e. the dose required to produce 50% reduction in specific binding[7,13].

Counts measured within a brain region represent activity associated with: 1) binding to the receptor; 2) non-specific binding within the extracellular space; 3) free tracer; and 4) blood vessels traversing the region. Errors in calculation of drug potency or percentage receptor occupancy may result from inaccurate estimate of activity associated with radioligand receptor binding. One technique for estimating receptor-bound activity is to subtract the concentration of activity in a reference region devoid of receptors (non-specific uptake + free activity) from the concentration of total uptake in the region of interest (specific + non-specific uptake + free activity). This assumes equivalent non-specific and free uptake in the region of interest and the reference area. Some radioligands with wide distribution of receptors throughout brain, like the benzodiazepine receptor radioligand [^{123}I]iomazenil, do not have suitable reference regions of low specific uptake. In such cases, estimation of activity associated with specific receptor binding can be made by administering a receptor-saturating dose of displacing drug to determine within the region of interest the percentage of activity that is non-displaceable (i.e. non-specific activity) (Fig. 4). This is feasible in

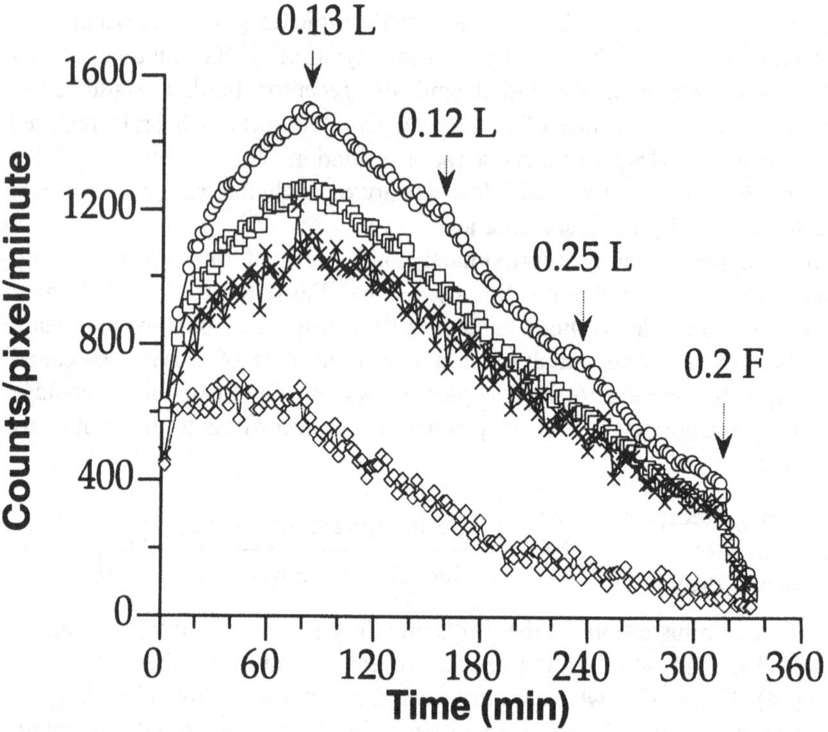

Fig. 4. Regional brain time–activity curves in various brain regions (O—occipital, □—temporoparietal, X—frontal, ◇—striatum) in baboon following the bolus injection of the benzodiazepine receptor agent [^{123}I]iomazenil. Arrows indicate administration of three doses of lorazepam 'L' (0.13, 0.12 and 0.25 mg/kg i.v.) and a final dose of the BZ antagonist flumazenil 'F' (0.2 mg/kg i.v.). Lorazepam enhances the rate of washout of cortical activity. An ED_{50}, or the dose required to produce 50% reduction in cortical activity, provides an in vivo measure of drug potency.

animal experiments but may not be possible in human SPET studies where the high doses of pharmacologically active agents needed to produce complete displacement from receptor sites may be associated with untoward side effects.

Displacement of brain activity requires doses of displacing drug sufficient to occupy a significant proportion of binding sites. Antipsychotics are clinically effective at relatively high percentage receptor occupancies[11]; hence, standard clinical doses of antipsychotic cause displacement of radiotracer bound to dopamine receptors. Other psychotropic agents, like the benzodiazepines, are clinically effective at low percentage receptor occupancies. In this instance, administration of usual clinical doses of benzodiazepines during dynamic SPET imaging of BZ receptors with [^{123}I]iomazenil produce no measurable effect on regional brain activity until much higher doses are administered[13].

Some agents like D-amphetamine, a potent releaser of endogenous dopamine, may produce displacement of brain activity associated wtih binding to dopamine receptors by indirect means. D-Amphetamine is a potent releaser of endogenous dopamine from the presynaptic neurone into the synapse. The increased intrasynaptic dopamine may compete for binding with radiotracer bound to postsynaptic dopamine receptors[7]. Hence, amphetamine-induced displacement is related to the amount of dopamine released rather than direct effects of amphetamine at the binding site.

Factors affecting displacement of receptor-bound radioligand by drugs competing either directly or indirectly for receptor binding include properties of the radioligand such as lipophilicity and receptor affinity and the characteristics of the displacing drug like rate of peripheral clearance, ease of penetrance into brain and affinity for the target receptor.

Displacement of the radioligand from the receptor occurs following tracer dissociation from receptors, binding of the competing drug to available sites and the diffusion of radiotracer from the vicinity of the receptor. For radiotracers which are reversibly bound, association and dissociation from receptors is a dynamic process. The frequency with which tracer associates and dissociates from the binding site determines the amount of time a site will be available for binding by the displacing drug. Once the radioligand has dissociated from the receptor, the ease with which it leaves the synaptic region determines the probability of again associating with an available receptor. This is partly a function of the lipophilicity of the radioligand. The greater the lipophilicity of the tracer, the more rapid the egress from the synaptic region and return to the periphery.

The properties of displacing drug affecting its ability to displace radioligand from binding sites include the rate of peripheral clearance, ease of penetrance across the blood–brain barrier and affinity for the target receptor. Agents which are rapidly metabolized to inactive metabolites, demonstrate poor penetrance of the blood–brain barrier or have fast receptor off rates with rapid diffusion out of the synaptic region, will be less effective displacers of radioligand binding from receptors. Non-specific effects of the displacing drug may be a potential confound to interpreting patterns of brain activity washout. If the displacing drug also increases brain blood flow, radiotracer will wash out faster from brain.

A potential source of error in the analysis of percentage receptor occupancy is the problem of discriminating the effects of the displacing drug from the normal washout of tracer from a brain region. High between-subject variability in the rate of peripheral clearance of tracer, hepatic metabolism, plasma protein binding, renal perfusion, in addition to differ-

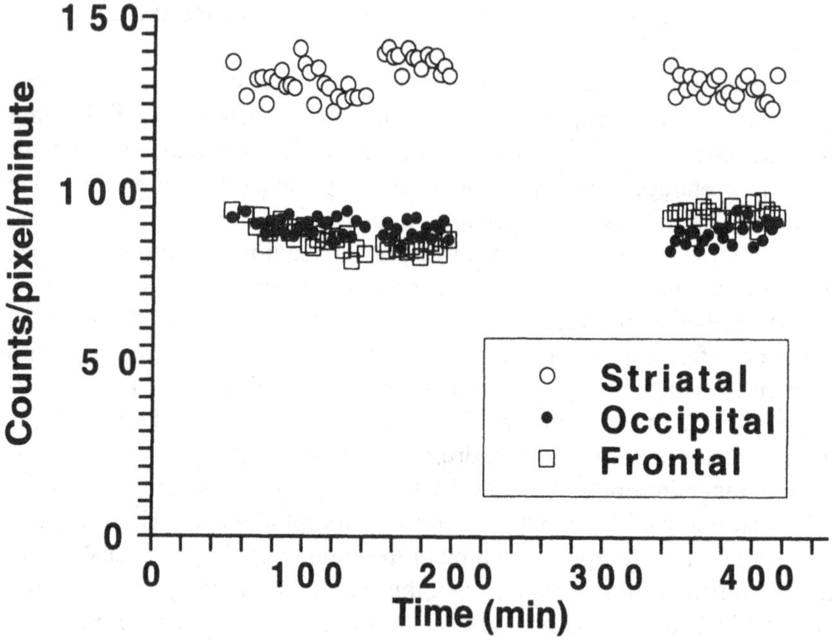

Fig. 5. Dynamic SPET data from a healthy human subject receiving a bolus plus constant infusion of [^{123}I]IBZM. All regions sampled demonstrate unchanging time–activity data over the course of the examination suggesting that an equilibrium condition has been attained.

ences in receptor density, contributes to this variability. It is possible to correct for the rate of tracer washout within a subject by obtaining a baseline study[13], but this assumes brain washout rates are identical on the two test days. Another solution to this problem is to deliver the radioligand as a continuous infusion. With this paradigm there is eventually achieved an unchanging time–activity curve against which the effects of displacing drugs may be evaluated (Figs 5, 6).

Within-scan drug displacement techniques improve the reliability of sampling within the same brain region pre- and post-test drug injection. Protocols requiring baseline and treatment scans may suffer from errors in precise region of interest placement under test–retest conditions. Within-scan methods have been used in the estimation of receptor occupancy of benzodiazepines and antipsychotic agents in animals and humans (Figs 4, 6).

Finally, accurate estimation of receptor occupancy by psychotropic drugs requires a linearity between detected counts and actual radioactivity over the range of measurements in the SPET experiment. At high count rates, gamma cameras exhibit decreasing efficiency, referred to as dead-time

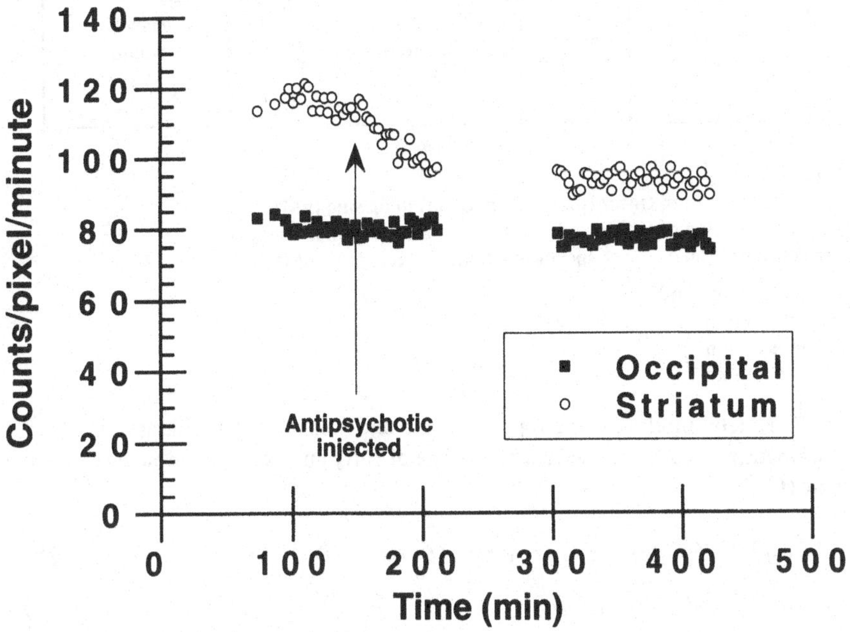

Fig. 6. Dynamic SPET time–activity data in occipital cortex and striatum in a healthy human subject administered [^{123}I]IBZM as a continuous tracer infusion over 7 h. At the arrow the subject received an intravenous injection of a dopamine antagonist. Note displacement of activity from striatum, a region rich in dopamine receptors with no effect in receptor-poor occipital cortex.

effect. Most SPET tomographs demonstrate good linearity over the range of activity encountered in neuroreceptor studies.

Approaches to quantitating receptor number

Kinetic modelling of SPET data Recently, kinetic modelling of tracer uptake and washout has been applied to animal and human SPET time–activity data[8,9]. For these analyses a model is constructed to describe the transfer of activity between compartments; blood (C_1), non-specific brain uptake (including free tracer within the extracellular space) (C_2) and activity bound to the target receptor (C_3) (Fig. 7). The model is characterized by a set of differential equations which describe the concentration of free parent radiotracer in blood and the two brain compartments as a function of time. The three-compartment, four-parameter kinetic model of tracer movement into brain assumes first-order kinetic processes. Activity within each compartment at time t is described by the following:

$$dC_{1(t)}/dt = k_2C_2(t) - K_1C_1(t) \qquad (2a)$$

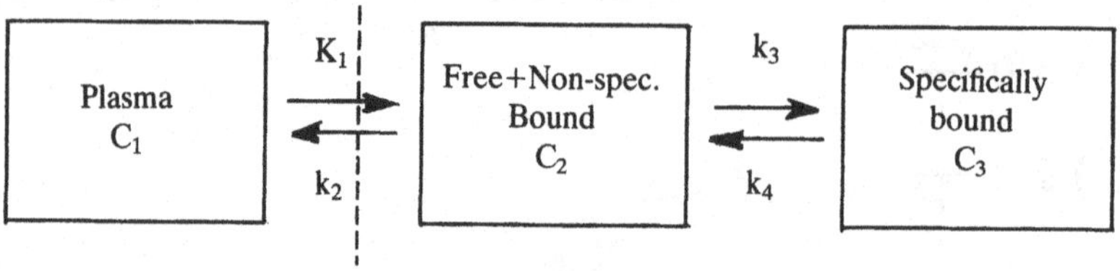

where
C_1 = concentration of tracer (parent compound) in plasma (nM)
C_2 = concentration of free ligand + non-specifically bound in brain (nM)
C_3 = concentration of tracer specifically bound to receptor (nM)

K_1 = units of ml min^{-1}
k_2 = units of min^{-1}
k_3 = units of min^{-1}
k_4 = units of min^{-1}

Fig. 7. Kinetic model describing the uptake and washout of radiotracer in brain. The kinetic rate constants determine the rate of entry and egress from each compartment ($C_{1\text{-}3}$).

$$dC_{2(t)}/dt = K_1C_1(t) - k_2C_2(t) + k_4C_3(t) - k_3C_2(t) \tag{2b}$$

$$dC_{3(t)}/dt = k_3C_2(t) - k_4C_3(t) \tag{2c}$$

A regional brain binding potential equal to the density of receptors divided by the inverse binding affinity (B_{max}/K_d) may be calculated from data acquired within a single SPET scanning session. This technique requires acquisition of serial brain images (constituting non-specific brain C_2, and receptor-bound C_3 compartments) and concomitant determination of arterialfree parent compound (blood compartment, C_1). Data is converted into absolute concentration of activity (nC_i/cc) in brain and blood (nC_i/ml) for computer fitting of the experimental data to the compartmental model using an iterative least squares minimization procedure[14–16]. The computer fit provides the kinetic transfer coefficients (Fig. 8) K_1, k_2, k_3 and k_4. At high activity, where receptor occupancy is negligible ($B < B_{max}$), the binding potential is related to the model parameters by the equation:

$$B.P. = \frac{K_1k_3}{f_1k_2k_4} \tag{3}$$

Equilibrium methods using continuous infusions of radiotracer The transfer of activity between compartments in the kinetic method are described by coupled differential equations (Eqns (2a)–(2c)). If the rate of change of activity between compartments is zero, the differential equations simplify to trivial algebraic solutions. Equilibration of tracer within brain may be obtained by administering radioligand as a continuous infusion. When brain activity is unchanging and is expressed as parent radiotracer bound to receptors, the ratio of the specifically bound activity (B_e) to free ligand (F) within brain is equal to the binding potential, B_{max}/K_d.

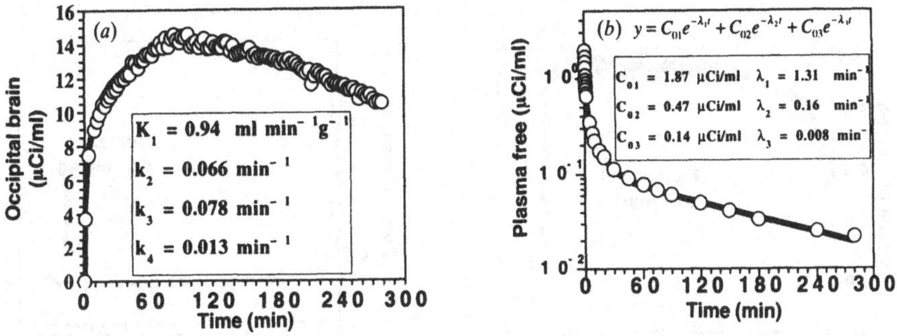

Fig. 8. [^{123}I]Iomazenil study in monkey cortex and arterial plasma following a single bolus of radiotracer. Brain (*a*) and plasma (*b*) time–activity curves in a baboon after intravenous administration of a single dose of [^{123}I]iomazenil fit to an unconstrained three-compartment, four-parameter kinetic model. Inset in panel (*a*) shows rate constants derived from compartmental analysis of the data. Inset in panel (*b*) shows the plasma parameters from a least squares fit to a 3-exponential arterial input function.

At equilibrium, the concentration of receptor-bound ligand (B_e) is given by

$$B_e = \frac{B_{\max} F}{K_d + F} \tag{4}$$

where F is the concentration of free ligand in brain. Rearranging this equation gives

$$\frac{B_e}{F} = \frac{B_{\max} - B_e}{K_d} \approx \frac{B_{\max}}{K_d} = \text{B.P.} \quad \text{At high specific activity } (B_e << B_{\max}). \tag{5}$$

Continuous infusion methods eliminate variability in cortical uptake and distribution of tracer due to differences in blood flow alone because at equilibrium free parent compound in brain and plasma are equal and unchanging. Thus, a single measurement of the receptor-bound concentration of receptor-bound tracer (B_e) and free tracer (F) will give the binding potential.

Referring to Fig. 7, if equilibrium conditions are met, the free level in the brain (f_2C_2) will equal the free level in the plasma (f_1C_1), where f_1 and f_2 are the fraction of free tracer within plasma and brain compartments, respectively. Specifically bound tracer can be derived from the total concentration measured by the SPECT image (C_{TOTAL}) as follows. Given that:

$$C_{\text{TOTAL}} = C_2 + C_3, \tag{6}$$

$$C_3 = B_e$$

$$f_1C_1 = f_2C_2 \quad \text{or} \quad C_2 = \frac{f_1C_1}{f_2} \tag{7}$$

Substituting,

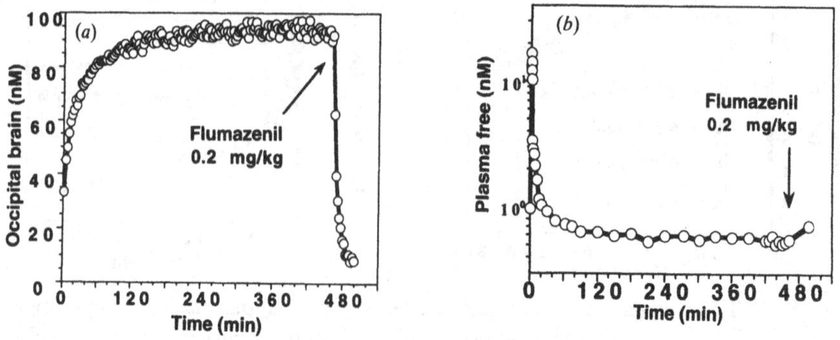

Fig. 9. Occipital activity (*a*) and plasma parent tracer (*b*) following the administration of [^{123}I]iomazenil as a bolus followed by continuous infusion. This method produces unchanging levels of brain activity consistent with achievement of equilibration of association: dissociation of radiotracer binding to BZ receptors. A receptor saturating dose of flumazenil (0.2 mg/kg i.v.) was administered at the end of the dynamic study to demonstrate the extent of [^{123}I]iomazenil bound to BZ receptors.

$$C_{\text{TOTAL}} = \frac{f_1 C_1}{f_2} + B_e \quad \text{or} \quad B_e = C_{\text{TOTAL}} - \frac{f_1 C_1}{f_2} \tag{8}$$

The plasma-free fraction f_1 (free parent compound not protein bound) and concentration C_1 are measured directly in the experiment. The free fraction in brain, f_2, is taken from the mean value derived in kinetic experiments. Thus, it is possible to utilize regional brain count data from a scan after equilibration has been achieved and a blood measurement (which is equal to the free parent compound in brain) to calculate a ratio of specific: non-specific activity equal to binding potential. Fig. 9 illustrates the achievement of equilibrium in a monkey receiving a bolus plus constant infusion of [^{123}I]iomazenil.

The term 'equilibrium' may refer to either a true equilibrium or transient equilibrium. True equilibrium or peak equilibrium[17] occurs at the time of peak specific uptake, i.e. when the differential of the specific activity curve relative to time is zero[18]. Transient equilibrium[19], also referred to as constant ratio, secular equilibrium[18] or pseudo-equilibrium, denotes a constant ratio of tissue to plasma or target to background regions within an organ.

During constant infusion studies the body as a whole may be described as a steady state in which the rate of tracer delivery equals the rate of clearance of parent tracer from the plasma. This steady state provides a constant level of parent tracer in plasma – even in the face of increasing total plasma activity caused by the accumulation of radiometabolites. In the brain, the constant infusion results in stable levels of total striatal activity, total occipital activity and specific striatal uptake. In contrast to plasma, levels of both parent tracer and total radioactivity are constant. Differences between brain and plasma are due to the fact that for many SPET neuroreceptor agents radiolabelled metabolites do not cross the blood–brain barrier[20]. In this instance the terms 'true equilibrium' and 'constant ratio' would both apply with the former representing the more stringent equilibrium condition.

In contrast to imaging studies, the homogenate binding literature defines equilibrium as a dynamic, reversible state in which the rate of ligand association equals its rate of dissociation[21]. This definition may also apply to the SPET neuroreceptor studies involving administration of tracer as a continuous infusion when the binding of tracer is reversible. In view of the reversibility of tracer binding and constant levels of brain activity and free parent tracer in plasma, the constant infusion of radiotracer is presumed to result in a state in which the free level of tracer in the vicinity of the receptor is constant; the tracer is dynamically binding and rebinding; the rates of association and dissociation are equal.

Truly quantitative SPET methods like kinetic modelling of time–activity data or equilibrium measurements require accurate recovery of emitted photons. Several physical factors previously mentioned are obstacles to converting regional brain counts measured with SPET tomographs into absolute units of activity. These factors include scattering of photons traversing brain tissue, inhomogeneous absorption of photons in different tissue densities and poor counting statistics encountered in studies requiring rapid, dynamic SPET acquisitions[22].

Scattered photons lose energy and change direction degrading image resolution and contaminating measurement of photons within the characteristic energy peak of the isotope. For example, [^{123}I]-labelled tracers have 4% high energy emissions that 'spill down' into the reconstruction window adding counts to the estimate.

Photons travelling through matter are attenuated as a function of the density and thickness of the attenuating medium. Medium energy photons from [^{99m}Tc] and [^{123}I] (140 keV and 159 keV, respectively) emanating from structures deep within brain undergo significant attenuation. Most brain SPET algorithms employ a linear attenuation correction based on an ellipse placed around brain and assuming uniform brain attenuation equal to water. Such a method does not correct for inhomogeneity of attentuation based on variability in skull thickness or brain tissue densities (Table 2).

Characteristics of SPET neuroreceptor agents

The selection of the appropriate outcome measure for analysis of brain SPET data depends to a large extent on the properties of the radiotracer. Ideally, SPET radioligands are stable in vivo, readily cross the blood–brain barrier, have high affinity and selectivity for the receptor site, bind reversibly, have low non-specific brain uptake and are free of active metabolites that cross the blood–brain barrier and compete with parent compound for

Table 2.

SPET measure	Advantage	Disadvantage
Ratio target to reference region	• Simplicity • No blood sampling • Corrects for many between-scan sources of variability	• Not linearly releated to receptor density • Affected by differences in peripheral clearance of tracer
Time–activity curve analyses	• Simplicity • No blood sampling	• Not linearly related to receptor density • Affected by differences in peripheral clearance of tracer, region of interest size
Kinetic modelling	• Provides measure of blood flow and receptor binding potential which is linearly related to receptor density	• Necessity of arterial sampling • Requires accurate recovery of photons including scatter and attenuation correction to express data as absolute activity
Equilibrium method	• Provides measure linearly related to receptor density	• Requires at least venous sampling • Long infusion time (hours) required • Requires accurate recovery of photons including scatter and attenuation correction to express data as absolute activity

receptor binding. Tracers that exhibit rapid brain uptake and washout phases within a scanning session are more easily modelled using kinetic methods described above than radioligands with little demonstrable washout during the SPET scan.

An example of a radioligand with very slow brain washout after bolus administration is the monoamine transporter ligand [^{123}I]β-CIT, alternatively designated RTI-55[23–25]. Following bolus injection in healthy human subjects, activity within the striatum increases until a plateau is reached

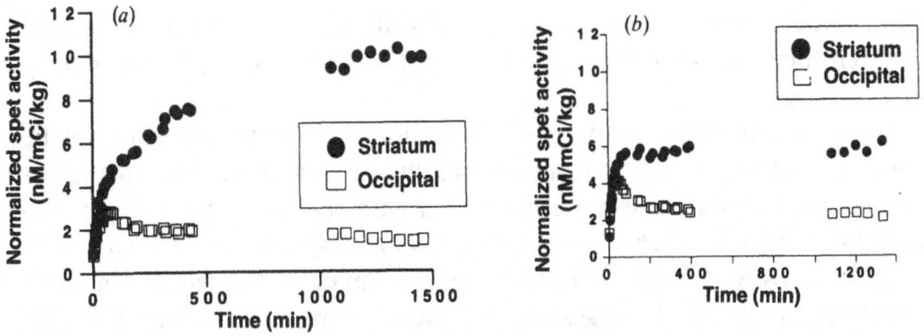

Fig. 10. Time–activity data acquired over 24 h period in a healthy subject (*a*) and patient with idiopathic Parkinson's disease (*b*) receiving a bolus injection of [¹²³I]β-CIT. Note increasing striatal activity over the first 1000 min after tracer injection, while occipital cortex attains peak levels within first hour of tracer injection then reaches a plateau where tracer is washing out at very slow rates. Very slow washout rates in striatum and occipital cortex are due to exceedingly long clearance times of the free parent tracer from the plasma pool. Patient shows earlier time to peak uptake with plateau at lower level of activity.

approximately 18–24 h post-[¹²³I]β-CIT administration. SPET examinations in idiopathic Parkinson's disease (PD) patients provide an instructive comparison to the healthy subjects. PD is associated with pathophysiological loss of dopamine transporters[26,27] located on dopamine-producing nigral neurones projecting to striatum[28]. Dynamic SPET measurements in Parkinson's disease exhibit shorter times to peak activity and plateau within striatum (Fig. 10) as would be expected by pharmacokinetic theory. For tracers with protracted uptake and extremely slow brain washout, rates like [¹²³I]β-CIT kinetic modelling approaches are troublesome to apply. When there is very slow washout (i.e. k_4 is small, but not zero), accurate determination of the transfer coefficients are very sensitive to noise. On the other hand, ratio analyses are relatively robust and stable for long periods after injection. The fact that activity levels are changing so slowly in brain regions provides a relatively constant ratio similar to the conditions achieved during bolus plus continuous infusion methods in other radioligands.

The quality of quantitative and semi-quantitative analyses of receptor binding depends on the radioligand selectivity for the targeted receptor, the extent of non-specific brain uptake and the density of binding sites in regional brain. Few radioligands demonstrate complete selectivity for individual receptor subtypes. The iodinated benzamide compounds [¹²³I]-IBZM and [¹²³I]IBF are potent at both dopamine D_2 and D_3 receptors while [¹²³I]β-CIT binds to dopamine, serotonin and norepinephrine transporters. This may be less a factor if there is a high degree of heterogeneity in the brain distribution of the different receptors. This is the case of [¹²³I]β-CIT, where, due to the much larger proportion of striatal dopamine compared with serotonin transporters, the SPET signal in this region represents mainly DA binding.

If the density of receptors within a brain region is low, it may not be possible to obtain accurate data reflecting the density of binding sites. Considered another way, the noise associated with the signal for radioligands with low target to background activity ratios may obscure evaluation of receptor density. [^{123}I]IBF produces higher target to background activity levels than [^{123}I]IBZM suggesting, all other factors being equal, that this ligand will be superior to [^{123}I]IBZM for quantitating regional brain receptor distribution. [^{123}I]epidepride and related compounds are additional examples of high affinity agents with high striatal target to background ratios[29]. Since cortical dopamine D_2 receptors are less densely distributed by a factor of 100 compared with striatum, examination of dopamine receptors in extrastriatal regions requires extremely high specific:non-specific binding levels.

Conclusions

Neuroreceptor SPET is a useful tool for studying alterations of receptors in neuropsychiatric illness and characterizing in vivo effects of psychotropic medications or drugs of abuse. Improvements in instrumentation and techniques for enhancing accurate recovery of activity as well as development of new radiochemical probes will be pivotal in future SPET work.

Improved quantitation with SPET will require more accurate correction for attentuated and scattered photons[30]. Transmission maps for attenuation correction of SPET data have been utilized, including methods which acquire the transmission and emission data simultaneously, thus obviating problems of subject realignment between scans. The contribution of scattered photons to counts measured within the photopeak data window has been estimated by a number of techniques, including reconstructing images using split, asymmetric energy windows. Some of these methods reduce the counts within the reconstruction window and may require longer imaging times and thus result in poorer temporal resolution of the time–activity data during dynamic SPET studies. Improvements of the energy resolution of SPET instruments will help in more accurate approximations of scatter effects.

The frequently encountered compromise between spatial resolution and camera sensitivity suggests an area for instrumentation improvement. Collimators which provide high spatial resolution may be of such poor sensitivity to limit frequent sampling during dynamic SPET studies. Advances in collimation and camera design will continue to produce improvement in spatial resolution with limited penalty in sensitivity.

Further refinement of SPET neuroreceptor agents will address issues of improved selectivity, greater target to background uptake and idealized kinetic properties for selected outcome measures. In addition, the production of new ligands with selectivity for other receptor systems, including serotonergic and glutaminergic binding sites, will be crucial tools for investigating pathophysiologial hypotheses of neuropsychiatric illness in living human brain.

In summary, neuroreceptor SPET is a powerful, if nascent, tool for the in vivo examination of brain receptor function. SPET measurement of the in vivo properties of labelled drug and dose–response occupancy of target receptors make neuroreceptor SPET particularly suited to new drug development.

Acknowledgements
This work was supported by the Schizophrenia Biological Research Center of the West Haven VAMC. The author gratefully acknowledges the helpful comments of Drs Robert Innis and Paul Hoffer.

References

(1) Kuhl D. Rotational scanning of the liver. *Radiology* 1958.
(2) Innis R. Neuroreceptor imaging with SPECT. *J Clin Psychiat* 1992; 53 (suppl): 29–34.
(3) Sikoloff L. Relationships among local functional activity, energy metabolism, and blood flow in the central nervous system. *Fed Proc* 1981; 40: 2311.
(4) Woods S, Hegeman I, Zubal IG et al. Visual stimulation increases technetium-[^{99m}]-HMPAO distribution in human visual cortex. *J Nucl Med* 1991; 32: 210–15.
(5) Pilowsky L, Costa D, Ell PJ, Murray RM, Verhoeff NPLG, Kerwin RW. Clozapine, single photon emission tomography, and the D2 dopamine receptor blockade hypothesis of schizophrenia. *Lancet* 1992; 340: 199–202.
(6) Seibyl J, Woods S, Zoghbi SS et al. Dynamic SPECT imaging of dopamine D2 receptors in human subjects with [^{123}I]IBZM. *J Nucl Med* 1992; 33: 1964–71.
(7) Innis R, Al-Tikriti M, Zoghbi S et al. SPECT imaging of the benzodiazepine receptor: feasibility of in vivo potency measurements from stepwise displacement curves. *J Nucl Med* 1991; 32: 1754–61.
(8) Abi-Dargham A, Laruelle M, Seibyl J et al. SPECT measurements of benzodiazepine receptors in human brain with [^{123}I]iomazenil: kinetic and equilibrium paradigms. *J Nucl Med* 1994; 35: 228–38.
(9) Laruelle M, Baldwin R, Rattner Z et al. SPECT quantification of [^{123}I]iomazenil binding to benzodiazepine receptors in nonhuman primates. I. Kinetic modeling of single bolus experiments. *J Cereb Blood Flow Metab* 1994; 14: 439–52.
(10) Woods S, Seibyl J, Goddard A et et. Dynamic SPECT imaging after injection of the benzodiazepine receptor ligand [123-I]iomazenil in healthy human subjects. *Psychiat Res* 1992; 45: 67–77.
(11) Farde L, Nordström A, Wiesel F, Pauli S, Halldin C, Sedvall G. Positron

emission tomographic analysis of central D1 and D2 dopamine receptor occupancy in patients treated with classical neuroleptics and clozapine: relation to extrapyramidal side effects. *Arch Gen Psychiat* 1992; 49: 538–44.
(12) Nordström A, Farde L, Wiesel FA et al. D2-dopamine receptor occupancy in relation to antipsychotic drug effects: a double-blind PET study of schizophrenic patients. *Biol Psychiat* 1993; 33: 227–35.
(13) Sybirska E, Seibyl J, Bremner J et al. [^{123}I] iomazenil SPECT imaging demonstrates significant benzodiazepine receptor reserve in human and nonhuman primate brain. *Neuropharmacology* 1993; 32: 671–80.
(14) Logan J, Wolf AP, Shiue C-Y, Fowler JS. Kinetic modeling of receptor ligand binding applied to positron emission tomography studies with neuroleptic tracers. *J Neurochem* 1987; 48: 73–83.
(15) Frost JJ, Douglass KH, Mayberg HS et al. Multicompartmental analysis of [^{11}C]carfentanil binding to opiate receptors in humans measured by positron emission tomography. *J Cereb Blood Flow Metab* 1989; 9: 398–409.
(16) Sadzot B, Price JC, Mayberg HS et al. Quantification of human opiate receptor concentration and affinity using high and low specific activity [^{11}C]diprenorphine and positron emission tomography. *J Cereb Blood Flow Metab* 1991; 11: 204–19.
(17) Savic I, Roland P, Sedvall G, Persson A, Pauli S, Widen L. In vivo demonstration of reduced benzodiazepine receptor binding in human epileptic foci. *Lancet* 1988; 2: 863–6.
(18) Farde L, Eriksson L, Blomquist G, Halldin C. Kinetic analysis of central [^{11}C]raclopride binding to D2 dopamine receptors studies with PET – a comparison to the equilibrium analysis. *J Cereb Blood Flow Metab* 1989; 9: 696–708.
(19) Carson R, Channing M, Blasberg R et al. Comparison of bolus and infusion methods for receptor quantitation: application to [^{18}F]cyclofoxy and positron emission tomography. *J Cereb Blood Flow Metab* 1993; 13: 24–42.
(20) Kung H, Alavi A, Chang W et al. In vivo SPECT imaging of CNS D-2 dopamine receptors: initial studies with iodine [^{123}I]IBZM in humans. *J Nucl Med* 1990; 31: 573–9.
(21) Bylund D, Yamamura H. Methods for receptor binding. In: Yamamura HES, Kuhar M, eds. *Methods in neuroreceptor receptor analysis.* New York: Raven Press; 1990: 1–35.
(22) Lee K. *Computers in nuclear medicine: a practical approach.* New York: Society of Nuclear Medicine; 1991: 207–20.
(23) Madras BK, Spealman RD, Fahey MA, Neumeyer JL, Saha JK, Milius RA. Cocaine receptors labeled by [3H]-2β-carbomethoxy-3β-(4-fluorophenyl) tropane. *Mol Pharmacol* 1989; 36: 518–24.
(24) Boja JW, Patel A, Carroll FI et al. [^{125}I]RTI-55: a potent ligand for dopamine transporters. *Eur J Pharmacol* 1991; 194: 133–4.
(25) Laruelle M, Baldwin R, Malison R et al. SPECT imaging of dopamine and serotonin transporters with [^{123}I]β-CIT: pharmacological characterization of brain uptake in nonhuman primates. *Synapse* 1993; 13: 295–309.
(26) Niznik HB, Fogel E, Fassos FF, Seeman P. The dopamine transporter is absent in parkinsonian putamen and reduced in the caudate nucleus. *J Neurochem* 1991; 56: 192–8.

(27) Kaufman M, Madras B. Severe depletion of cocaine recognition sites associated with the dopamine transporter in Parkinson's-diseased striatum. *Synapse* 1991; 9: 43–9.

(28) Innis R, Seibyl J, Scanley B et al. SPECT imaging demonstrates loss of striatal monoamine transporters in Parkinson's disease. *PNAS* 1993; 90: 11965–9.

(29) Kessler RM, Votaw J, Schmidt DE et al. High affinity dopamine D2 receptor radioligands. 3. [^{123}I] and [^{125}I]epidepride: in vivo studies in rhesus monkey brain and comparison with in vitro pharmacokinetics in rat brain. *Life Sci* 1993; 53: 241–50.

(30) Blokland J, Reiber J, Pauwels E. Quantitative analysis in single photon emission computed tomography. *Eur J Nucl Med* 1992; 19: 47–61.

SPET blood flow studies and the functional anatomy of psychiatric disorders

G F BUSATTO

Functional imaging measures of blood flow and metabolism have become the most reliable and direct means to assess regional brain function in vivo and identify sites of dysfunction in a variety of neuropsychiatric disorders.

The sophisticated positron emission tomography (PET) technique continues to be the gold standard to perform those measurements. However, recent developments of the cheaper and more accessible single photon emission tomography (SPET) technique, including new SPET blood flow tracers and brain dedicated systems, have raised its quality to levels comparable to those of PET. This has not only enabled previous PET findings to be investigated in large samples, but also awarded SPET the status of a powerful tool in its own right to generate and test hypotheses about the pathophysiology and management of psychiatric disorders.

This chapter will evaluate the advances of modern SPET blood flow technology and review the most recent SPET studies on relevant psychiatric disorders, relating them to findings of other imaging modalities and current pathophysiological theories for the disorders in question.

Blood flow and its relationship to cerebral function

More than 100 years ago, after a series of rudimentary laboratory experiments with dogs, Roy and Sherrington[1] put forward the idea that regulatory mechanisms in the brain modify the supply of blood to specific areas in response to variations of levels of functional activity.

With the introduction of tracer methods to map cerebral blood flow (CBF) in vivo[2], an uncountable number of studies provided experimental confirmation to Roy and Sherrington's proposition[3–6], showing global and

All correspondence to: Dr G F Busatto, Section of Clinical Neuropharmacology, Department of Psychological Medicine, Institute of Psychiatry, De Crespigny Park, Denmark Hill, London SE5 8AF, UK.

Cambridge Medical Reviews: Neurobiology and Psychiatry Volume 3

regional blood flow changes in association with increases in functional activity.

Given that cerebral function is basically supported by oxidative metabolism and neither oxygen nor glucose can be stored in the brain, it is believed that regional increases in blood flow are meant to supply those substrates locally[7]. This notion has been first supported by quantitative autoradiographic studies of glucose utilization in animals[8] as well as in vivo studies showing parallel decreases in blood flow and energy metabolism in laboratory animals and humans anaesthetized with barbiturates[7,9]. Subsequent confirmation has come from PET studies which have demonstrated the existence of a tight coupling between regional blood flow and both glucose metabolism and oxygen consumption in most conditions[10,11].

In vivo tracer techniques to measure brain blood flow

The first in vivo method for measuring CBF was proposed by Kety and Schmidt in 1948[2]. Adapting Fick's principle for calculating cardiac output from arterial–venous differences in O_2 and CO_2 concentration, they were able to obtain values for whole-brain blood flow from the differences in the amount of the inert gas nitrous oxide in a peripheric artery and the jugular vein. This simple paradigm has become the basis for all subsequent in vivo methods for assessing blood flow and metabolism.

Lassen, Ingvar and colleagues were the first to use Kety and Schmidt's principle to obtain *regional* indices of cerebral blood flow (rCBF)[12,13]. The technique involved the intracarotid bolus injection of a radioactive inert gas (^{85}Kr and later ^{133}Xe) and the recording of its clearance rate through monitoring the levels of photon emission by the use of an external radiation detector. This simple and inexpensive method had its invasiveness significantly reduced with the introduction of its inhalatory modification (^{133}Xe inhalation rCBF technique)[14], which is still widely used nowadays. Measures of ^{133}Xe clearance rates can provide absolute quantitation of rCBF, and the quick tracer washout enables the acquisition of several studies in one single session. The precision of this topographic technique to record regional photon emission is, however, limited by the low photon energy of ^{133}Xe and several sources of error, mainly contamination with photons originated from contralateral and extracerebral areas. Furthermore, the rapid tracer washout prevents assessment of rCBF to structures deeper than the more superficial cortical rim[15].

Three-dimensional imaging of blood flow and metabolism has only become possible with the advent of PET and SPET, both of which enable the conversion of photon-emitted energy into tomographic maps of regional activity. In PET, radiation detectors arranged around the head record the simultaneous arrival of pairs of photons emitted in opposite directions as the result of interactions between tracer-emitted positrons and electrons from the tissue. In SPET, simpler detectors encircling the head record the regional patterns of brain activity after the administration of photon-emitting tracers.

PET measurements afford high sensitivity and spatial resolution, and when arterial sampling of tracer concentration is performed, absolute quantification of either rCBF, glucose metabolism or oxygen consumption can be obtained. However, the complexity of the technique and the need for an on-site cyclotron to produce the short-lived tracers make it a highly expensive resource, restricted to only a few centres. Although less precise than PET, the relative simplicity of SPET blood flow techniques make them much more affordable, readily available and suitable for studying large samples.

Current state of SPET blood flow techniques

Blood flow SPET tracers

With the development of fast rotating systems with high sensitivity[16], it has become possible to adapt the ^{133}Xe inhalation rCBF technique to SPET imaging. Although less artefactual problems are present in comparison with the topographic technique, the rapid washout and poor imaging properties of ^{133}Xe still mitigate against high resolution imaging.

Several alternative compounds, with better physical properties in comparison with ^{133}Xe, have been developed[17]. These are invariably neutral, small and highly lipophilic molecules which quickly cross the blood–brain barrier through passive diffusion in proportion to blood flow[18]. They also have high extraction efficiency into the brain and retain a fixed distribution for long enough to allow reliable image acquisition[15].

N-Iso-propyl-[^{123}iodine]-p-iodoamphetamine (^{123}I-IMP) This was the first of the new SPET blood flow tracers to be made commercially available. After intravenous injection, it is rapidly taken up into the brain with high first-pass extraction efficiency[19]. Peak uptake is reached after 15 to 20 min, and involves an as yet unclear intracellular transformation into a non-lipophilic compound. The ^{123}I-IMP distribution remains relatively stable between 20 min and 1 h after injection, which is the ideal time gap for image acquisition[20]. After that, its regional distribution changes fairly quickly, and the proportionality to blood flow is lost.

Although ^{123}I-IMP fulfils the basic requirements of a suitable SPET blood perfusion tracer, its use is hampered by a series of limitations. A cyclotron is needed to produce ^{123}I, and the relatively short physical half-life of the isotope makes difficult its transport to the sites of use[21]. Thus, the tracer is not readily available, and usually advance ordering is needed. Moreover, the high photon energy of ^{123}I limits the radiation dose that can be administered and therefore prevents high resolution imaging[22].

Little data has been obtained with ^{123}I-IMP SPET in comparison with other functional imaging modalities, although comparisons with the ^{133}Xe inhalation rCBF technique suggest that the ^{123}I-IMP distribution in the brain is indeed proportional to blood flow in normal subjects[23]. This remains to be confirmed in diseased states.

Technetium-99m-hexamethylpropyleneamine oxime (^{99m}Tc-HMPAO)

^{99m}Tc-HMPAO has become the most widely used SPET tracer for rCBF measurements. Given in intravenous injection, it is quickly taken up into the brain with high extraction efficiency in proportion to blood flow[24]. Due to a glutathione-mediated transformation into a hydrophilic metabolite, the tracer gets intracellularly trapped after 2 to 3 min, and remains in a stable distribution for many hours[25]. This 'freeze-frame' picture of blood flow corresponding to the time of injection can therefore be imaged later, almost without loss of useful information. These properties make ^{99m}Tc-HMPAO particularly useful in the study of less cooperative patients, allowing time and care to be taken in preparing the patient for scanning and therefore improving his/her compliance with the procedure.

^{99m}Tc is produced by generator systems and delivered on a weekly basis to its sites of use, where ^{99m}Tc-HMPAO can be reconstituted using a commercially available kit. The radioligand is therefore cheap, can be stored for months and is available on a daily basis. After reconstitution, however, ^{99m}Tc-HMPAO is highly unstable in vitro; it is therefore recommended that administration be performed as soon as possible after reconstitution[15]. The shorter physical half-life time of ^{99m}Tc (6 h) compared with ^{123}I (13 h) and the emission of lower energy photons allows relatively larger radiation doses to be used with ^{99m}Tc-HMPAO, providing high resolution images or alternatively shortening the necessary imaging time.

The in vivo validation of ^{99m}Tc-HMPAO SPET has been conducted against rCBF PET[26,27] and the ^{133}Xe inhalation rCBF technique[28], and has demonstrated that ^{99m}Tc-HMPAO images correspond to blood flow in most situations. It is, however, known that underestimation of rCBF can occur with ^{99m}Tc-HMPAO SPET[27,29]. This is more prevalent in highly perfused areas, and is probably due to early back-diffusion out of the cells before trapping. An algorithm based on parallel ^{133}Xe imaging has been proposed to correct for that phenomenon[29], and has been used in some studies[30].

Technetium-99m-ethylcysteinate dimer (^{99m}Tc-ECD) Limited data is available on this recently developed SPET blood perfusion tracer. As with ^{99m}Tc-HMPAO, brain uptake is quick and tracer distribution stable for long periods. A few studies have been conducted comparing ^{99m}Tc-ECD and ^{99m}Tc-

HMPAO, most of them qualitatively only[31]. ^{99m}Tc-ECD SPET images seem to have quality comparable with that of ^{99m}Tc-HMPAO, and given the quick blood clearance of the tracer, background activity is low and image contrast said to be enhanced[21]. Also, ^{99m}Tc-ECD is stable in vitro, and its rapid urinary excretion reduces the amount of radiation to which subjects are exposed[21]. It has, however, been suggested that the usefulness of ^{99m}Tc-ECD may be hampered by the fact that, unlike with ^{99m}Tc-HMPAO, early washout from the brain can be high[32] and regionally variable[33].

The basic characteristics of the tracers mentioned above are summarized in Table 1.

SPET equipment

Single rotating gamma cameras used for conventional two-dimensional planar imaging can be adapted for tomographic single photon emission imaging. After tracer administration, the camera rotates around the subject acquiring sequential planar views of the head at equally spaced angles, which are later combined and reconstructed to provide a three-dimensional picture of rCBF[17]. However, sensitivity is limited and long imaging times are required. This has been overcome with the development of brain dedicated SPET systems. Typically, these are compact systems built with multiple detectors positioned in close proximity to the subject's head, improving dramatically the sensitivity of the device. As a result, high resolution brain SPET imaging is possible, with current equipment allowing for 6 to 9 mm resolution at full-width half-maximum (FWHM). Alternatively, scanning times can be significantly shortened, which is an important feature when less cooperative patients are to be studied.

The brain dedicated systems most frequently used in recent rCBF studies in psychiatry are: multiheaded gamma-camera systems; single-slice multidetector tomographs (Strichman Medical Equipment (SME) 810/900 systems); multislice multidetector tomographs (Tomomatic 32/64 systems, usable for ^{133}Xe SPET); and the recently developed high sensitivity, high resolution annular single-crystal brain imaging system (ASPECT). The physical characteristics and capabilities of these systems have been described[34–36].

Analysis of blood flow SPET data

With current SPET technology, full brain volume acquisitions can be reconstructed and displayed in any desired plane. Typically, images are displayed in transaxial, coronal and sagittal views.

Qualitative visual analysis of rCBF SPET images is highly informative in the investigation of organic brain disorders where gross functional changes are seen. However, in psychiatric syndromes where more subtle abnormalities are to be expected (such as schizophrenia and depression), the perform-

Table 1. *SPET tracers available for blood flow studies*

Tracer	Physical half-life	Administration	Usual dose	Advantages	Drawbacks
^{133}Xe	5 to 6 days	inhalatory or intravenous	110 to 250 MBq/litre or 350 to 750 MBq (i.v.)	– inexpensiveness – ready availability – absolute quantitation possible – multiple scans in one session possible	– poor physical properties – poor spatial resolution – high incidence of artefacts
^{123}I-IMP	13 hours	intravenous	110 to 185 MBq	– high brain uptake	– expensiveness – cyclotron needed – tracer not readily available – long half-life – radiation doses have to be limited – early tracer redistribution (1 h post-injection) – absolute quantitation not possible
^{99m}Tc-HMPAO	6 hours	intravenous	500 to 600 MBq	– inexpensiveness – ready availability – high brain uptake – distribution stable for several hours	– unstable in vitro – rCBF underestimation in highly perfused areas – absolute quantitation not possible
^{99m}Tc-ECD	6 hours	intravenous	500 to 600 MBq	– same as HMPAO *plus*: – rapid blood clearance – good image contrast – rapid renal excretion – low radiation exposure – high stability in vitro	– early washout from the brain – absolute quantitation not possible – limited data available to date

ance of some form of quantitative analysis is imperative. This usually involves the measurement of count estimates in regions of interest identified on selected slices. The placement of those regions is made either manually[37,38] or semi-automatically using predefined templates[39,40].

Although absolute quantitation of SPET data is theoretically possible with arterial sampling, the limitations of current methods for scatter and attenuation correction unfortunately prevent the acquisition of absolute quantitative measures of rCBF. Blood flow indices have therefore to be expressed in relative terms, with the count rates in each region of interest normalized to a reference measure. Usually, data is normalized to count rate estimates in the whole brain (or slice of interest), although normalization to reference regions (usually cerebellum or occipital cortex) is also frequently used. Neither method is free from drawbacks. Normalization to whole-brain measures influence the results by incorporating in the denominator regions that may be affected by blood flow abnormalities. On the other hand, the use of a reference region must assume that the same is spared by the disease process, which in many situations is difficult to predict. Clearly, more precise quantitation methods for SPET are needed.

Other developments in SPET data analysis have emerged. It has, for instance, become clear that the identification of regions of interest should be made with structural anatomical guidance, ideally with high spatial resolution magnetic resonance imaging (MRI) data from the same subject. This co-registration method, available for PET measurements[41], has now been applied with success to SPET imaging[42]. It not only improves the validity with which regions of interest are defined, but also enables the direct assessment of the relationship between rCBF indices and anatomical changes in diseased states.

Further improvements in rCBF PET data analysis are also potentially applicable to SPET. The method of statistical parametric mapping[43], used in several PET centres[44–47], allows image analysis and comparisons between groups to be made on a pixel by pixel basis, after stereotactic normalization. This exciting method avoids the imposition of predetermined regions of interest. Its application for rCBF SPET data analysis is desirable and foreseeable for the near future.

Variables that influence rCBF measurements

Measurements of rCBF are usually characterized by a high degree of random inter-subject variability. The effects of some of the potential sources of this variability have been assessed by several research groups.

Anxiety Although anxiety is a symptom frequently reported by subjects undergoing functional imaging procedures, the nature of its acute effects on blood flow patterns is probably complex and remains to be fully understood. Using the ^{133}Xe inhalation rCBF technique[48], Gur et al reported *increased* blood flow in association with anxiety in individuals who manifested low levels of that symptom during the imaging procedure; however, general *decreases* in rCBF were detected in subjects with high levels of anxiety. The authors suggested a curvilinear relationship between anxiety and metabolism, with high levels of anxiety associated with decreased metabolism. Reduced rCBF in association with anxiogenic stimulation has also been reported with simple phobic subjects[49] and patients with obsessive–compulsive disorder[50].

Possible specific regional effects of acute anxiety on blood flow patterns remain unclear. Increased activity in the temporal poles was some years ago described in association with anticipatory anxiety in normals in an rCBF PET study[51]. That finding has, however, been recently shown to be simply an artefact of temporalis muscle contraction[52]. More recently, a ^{99m}Tc-HMPAO study[53] reported reduced rCBF to temporal/occipital regions in phobic patients when listening to an anxiogenic exposure audio-tape.

Demographic variables A few studies have investigated the effects of gender differences on blood flow measures[54,55]. The results suggest that females have higher blood flow rates than males, which apparently are not accounted for by differences in blood viscosity or pressure between the sexes[54]. The reasons for those differences remain unclear.

rCBF reductions have been described in association with age[11,56], particularly in anterior regions. These have often been attributed to brain atrophy[7]. However, a recent PET study[57] has shown that age-related rCBF and oxygen consumption reductions, found in several cortical areas, are not exclusively dependent on the degree of brain atrophy as measured with computerized tomography (CT). The contribution of other factors to age-related rCBF reductions, such as diminished cellular metabolism or reduced neurotransmitter function, remain to be further elucidated.

Overall, the studies above highlight the need to carefully match subjects for age and sex when designing controlled studies using rCBF techniques.

In addition, ^{133}Xe inhalation rCBF studies[54] have found that the degree of lateralization of rCBF patterns measured during either verbal or spatial tasks is influenced by the subjects' hand preference patterns. Lateralized patterns of rCBF may also be found at rest, possibly in relation to the known anatomical asymmetries in the brain[7]. Matching subjects for handedness is therefore also advisable in rCBF studies, whether subjects are to be investigated at rest or during psychological activation.

Resting state and activation studies Metabolic indices are particularly subject to random variability when measured at rest[58], probably due to uncontrolled state factors such as level of wakefulness, attention to the environment and psychological activity during the scanning procedure[59,60]. In order to reduce that variability, the use of 'activation' paradigms (sensory, motor or cognitive tasks) that standardize the subjects' psychological state during rCBF and glucose metabolism measurements has been proposed and become widespread[60,61].

The potential of activation studies has been extended in the past few years. Tasks known to challenge specific regions of the brain have been used to try to unravel subtle deficits in those areas[60], or alternatively assess the reversibility of hypoactive patterns. Moreover, tasks that involve neuropsychological processes known to be abnormal in specific psychiatric syndromes have also been used during rCBF measurements, increasing the understanding of the pathophysiological mechanisms underlying those deficits[62]. Thus, Weinberger et al[59] used the inhalatory ^{133}Xe rCBF technique to study schizophrenic patients and normal controls at rest and during the Wisconsin Card Sorting Test (WCST), a cognitive task that invokes the engagement of the dorsolateral prefrontal cortex, and is known to be poorly performed by a substantial proportion of schizophrenic patients. While schizophrenics had marginal decreases in left dorsolateral prefrontal rCBF at rest, much more robust between-group differences emerged during the performance of the cognitive task.

Activation studies usually require the performance of multiple scans in the same session to allow comparisons of rCBF patterns during the challenging condition with rCBF at rest and/or during other control conditions. This is straightforward with rCBF PET or the ^{133}Xe inhalation rCBF technique, but not readily feasible with ^{99m}Tc-HMPAO and other SPET perfusion tracers. A recent advance has, however, been the development of split-dose SPET techniques[32,39,63], which enable two scans to be performed in one single session. The full tracer dose is divided in two injections, administered during a baseline condition and an activation condition, respectively. The second scan represents the superimposition of the rCBF distribution during the second injection upon the baseline distribution. Activation and baseline patterns are compared after the subtraction of the baseline counts from the second scan. Table 2 provides a list of recent controlled ^{99m}Tc-HMPAO rCBF SPET studies during psychological activation in different psychiatric populations.

Applications of SPET blood flow studies in psychiatric disorders

Research applications

Schizophrenia In the past few years, neurobiological research in psychiatry has concentrated more in schizophrenia than in any other disorder. Strong evidence of localized organic dysfunction has been gathered. Neuropathol-

Table 2. *Recent ^{99m}Tc-HMPAO SPET activation studies in psychiatry*

Study	Sample	Activation paradigm	Design	Scanner	Findings during activation condition
Rubin et al[30]	19 predominantly drug-naïve schizophrenics 12 normal volunteers	Wisconsin Card Sorting Test versus rest	split-dose technique	TOMOMATIC 232 multislice, multidetector system	decreased left inferior prefrontal rCBF and increased left striatal rCBF in patients
Lewis et al[62]	25 medicated schizophrenics 25 normal volunteers	verbal fluency task	single study with full ^{99m}Tc-HMPAO dose	SME 810 single-slice, multidetector system	decreased left frontal rCBF and increased temporo/occipital rCBF in patients
Busatto et al[64]	10 medicated schizophrenics 10 normal volunteers	recall of paired–associated words versus word repetition	split-dose technique	NEUROCAM (GE) triple-headed gamma-camera system	similar rCBF increases in medial temporal and other brain regions in both groups; increased rCBF in posterior cortical regions in patients
Kawasaki et al[65]	10 medicated schizophrenics 10 normal volunteers	Wisconsin Card Sorting Test versus rest	split-dose technique	TOSHIBA GCA9300A triple-headed gamma-camera system	decreased left and right medial prefrontal rCBF in patients
O'Carroll et al[53]	10 simple phobic patients	exposure audio-tape versus relaxation audio-tape	split-dose technique	SME 810 system	decreased right temporal and occipital rCBF
Moffoot et al[66]	18 patients with Korsakoff's psychosis divided in two groups	verbal fluency plus clonidine or saline infusion versus verbal fluency only	split-dose technique	SME 810 system	increased rCBF to anterior cingulate cortex during verbal fluency plus clonidine infusion only
Riddle et al[67]	10 patients with Alzheimer's disease 10 normal volunteers	recognition of words versus 'yes–no' repetition	split-dose technique	SME 810 system	increased prefrontal and anterior cingulate rCBF during activation in normals but not in patients; no between-group differences at baseline
Ebert et al[68]	6 medicated schizophrenics 6 medicated bipolar depressives 8 normal volunteers	somatosensory stimulation versus rest; volunteers studied at rest only	two scans 48 h apart	SIEMENS double-headed gamma-camera system	decreased left prefrontal rCBF in schizophrenics; decreased right inferior frontal rCBF in depressives

ogical studies have shown reduced weight of schizophrenic brains[69] as well as localized abnormalities implicating medial temporal, basal ganglia and frontal areas[70–72]. In vivo structural imaging with CT and MRI have shown enlarged ventricles in a large proportion of cases[73,74] as well as localized abnormalities, mainly in temporal areas[75,76].

Functional imaging studies have also contributed to the identification of foci of abnormal function in schizophrenia.

Using the ^{133}Xe intracarotid injection rCBF method, Ingvar and Franzén[77] were the first to report low anterior:posterior gradients of rCBF in chronic schizophrenia, as assessed by comparing the frontal:occipital rCBF ratios of schizophrenic patients and normal volunteers. This 'hypofrontal' pattern has been replicated in further ^{133}Xe inhalation rCBF studies[78,79] and extended with PET and SPET technology[80–87].

Although less consistently, functional abnormalities of the basal ganglia and related structures have also been reported in PET and SPET studies. Early et al[88] found increased rCBF to the left globus pallidus in a sample of never medicated schizophrenic patients. In contrast, PET studies have reported reduced ventral caudate metabolism in patients free from antipsychotics for at least 4 weeks[87,89]. It has been essential, in those studies, to restrict samples to unmedicated patients as increased striatal metabolism seems to be the most consistent rCBF effect of chronic antipsychotic use[90].

Consistent with structural imaging findings, temporal lobe changes have also been identified in some functional imaging studies, although not always in the same direction. Resting PET studies in the last decade reported both decreased[80] and increased temporal lobe glucose use[91] in chronic schizophrenics. High resolution PET instrumentation has now enabled the assessment of medially located temporal lobe structures, such as the hippocampus, with both hyperactivity[92] and hypoactivity[87,93] of that region having been reported very recently.

Thus, the functional imaging literature above converges on dysfunction of circuits involving frontal, striatal and temporal regions[90]. Several questions, however, remain to be answered. The relationship of regional dysfunction with schizophrenic symptoms, stage of disease and medication use is still unclear; both normal activity[94,95] and even 'hyperfrontal' patterns[96] have been described in acute unmedicated cases of schizophrenia. It is also unclear how the functional abnormalities relate to the neuropsychological deficits that underlie schizophrenic symptoms.

Taking advantage of recent technical improvements, rCBF SPET studies have helped to clarify some of those issues.

A recent ^{99m}Tc-HMPAO SPET study[97] examined rCBF at rest in 20 unmedicated, acutely ill schizophrenic patients compared with 20 matched controls. The main finding of the study was a pattern of 'hyperfrontality' in patients. This finding in a relatively large series of patients reinforces the idea that acute schizophrenic states may be associated with hyperactivity of the frontal lobes. In addition, correlations between schizophrenic symptoms and regional rCBF values were found. These included negative correlations between prefrontal cortex rCBF and negative symptom scores, and between left temporal rCBF and scores for delusions and hallucinations; positive correlations between formal thought disorder and anterior cingulate rCBF were also reported. These results support the notion that discrete patterns of rCBF underlie specific subsyndromes of schizophrenic symptoms, as first demonstrated in rCBF PET studies[98].

The characterization of brain activity patterns associated with specific schizophrenic symptoms has been further pursued in another recent ^{99m}Tc-HMPAO SPET study[99]. In a powerful test–retest design, 12 male medicated schizophrenic patients were investigated during and after the remission of psychotic episodes marked by auditory hallucinations. Significant rCBF increases in a frontal region encompassing Broca's area was found in the hallucinatory state as well as trends in the same direction in the left anterior cingulate and temporal cortex. The same areas are also known to be involved in normal language production and monitoring[100], supporting the view that hallucinatory phenomena in the disease is related to disturbances of those mental processes.

SPET cognitive activation paradigms have also been employed with schizophrenic patients. One split-dose ^{99m}Tc-HMPAO SPET study[30] investigated unmedicated patients (most of whom were drug naïve) during the WCST and replicated previous findings of 'hypofrontality'[59]. This finding supports the idea that the failure to activate prefrontal regions during challenging tasks is neither restricted to chronic patients nor is simply a correlate of the use of antipsychotics. Another case-control study using ^{99m}Tc-HMPAO SPET in a sample of 25 chronic schizophrenics[62] reported 'hypofrontal' blood flow in patients during a verbal fluency task which, as the WCST, demands integrity of prefrontal cortical regions to be adequately performed.

Our group has also employed activation paradigms in schizophrenia, with the purpose of investigating medial temporal functional abnormalities in the disease[64]. Using a split-dose ^{99m}Tc-HMPAO technique, we compared the patterns of rCBF in 10 chronic schizophrenic patients and 10 normal volunteers during a verbal memory task that effectively promoted rCBF increases to the left medial temporal region. Schizophrenic patients as a group did not fail to show increased rCBF to that region as predicted. However, other differences were found between the two groups, including distinct lateralized rCBF patterns and higher rCBF values in posterior cortical regions in schizophrenics. Further analysis of the data (unpublished results) showed that the latter finding contributed to a pattern of 'hypofrontality' (as assessed by anterior:posterior rCBF ratios) during the activation task in the patients' group.

Alzheimer's disease No neuropsychiatric disorder has had its regional patterns of brain function as well characterized as Alzheimer's disease (AD). Typical foci of hypoperfusion in temporo-parietal areas have been reported in rCBF SPET studies in a very high proportion of patients[101–104], confirming and extending earlier PET findings[105–107]. Other cortical areas, such as the frontal and occipital lobes, have also been implicated in severe cases, with subcortical regions generally being spared[108].

Correlations between rCBF deficits and performance on cognitive tests have also been investigated with SPET[102,109]. In general, hypoperfusion indices correlate with general measures of severity of cognitive deficits. Strong correlations between regional rCBF measures and specific cognitive deficits have also been reported, relating mainly language, praxis and memory impairments to temporal and parietal hypoperfusion[102,108,109].

The use of activation techniques has now enabled the assessment of the actual functional patterns *during* cognitive tasks known to be poorly performed by AD patients. A recent split-dose ^{99m}Tc-HMPAO SPET study[67] investigated rCBF changes associated with a recognition verbal memory task in 10 AD patients compared with normal volunteers. Significant frontal rCBF increases during the memory challenge were found in normals, a pattern that patients failed, as expected, to produce. Interestingly, however, instead of the typical perfusion deficits seen in resting studies in AD, no differences were found between the two groups during the baseline condition, where subjects were simply instructed to repeat 'yes' or 'no'. This suggests that activation of areas generally found to be hypoperfused in AD at rest can be obtained with non-demanding tasks, a finding also reported in ^{133}Xe rCBF[110] and PET[111] studies.

Activation studies with pharmacological challenges have also been performed in AD. Cholinergic challenges have been preferred, on the basis of both post-mortem neurochemical studies suggesting a relationship between severity of dementia and cholinergic dysfunction[112], and the clinical evidence that cholinergic enhancing drugs may bring some improvement to the cognitive performance of AD patients. Increase in ^{99m}Tc-HMPAO uptake in patients but not in normals after administration of the acetylcholinesterase inhibitor physostigmine has been reported[113], and seems to be particularly pronounced in left frontal regions[114]. Another acetylcholinesterase inhibitor, velnacrine, has also been shown to increase frontal cortical rCBF in AD patients[115]. Pharmacological activation studies seem, therefore, to be useful in providing information on the rCBF patterns underlying the effects of cholinergic agents in AD patients. The possible confounding effects of global CBF increases associated with cholinergic challenges have, however, not been fully elucidated.

The pathophysiological process responsible for the typical focal metabolic alterations in AD has not yet been clarified. The rCBF increases found in some activation studies suggest that the hypoperfusion deficits seen in the disease may be partially reversible[111], arguing against the idea that the blood flow deficits in AD may be simply correlates of neuronal loss. Alternatively, molecular neuropathology studies in AD have shown dysfunction of mitochondrial structures, suggesting that defects in the cell metabolic machinery could underlie the rCBF deficits[112]. Recently demonstrated correlations between post-mortem synaptic density and ante-mortem levels of cognitive impairment in AD[116] suggest that synaptic loss may also be a correlate of metabolic hypofunction in the disease.

Obsessive–compulsive disorder PET studies in obsessive–compulsive disorder (OCD) have suggested a role for cortical dysfunction in the disease, characterized mainly by excessive functional activity in orbital portions of the frontal lobes[117–119].

Recent SPET studies have extended those findings. Increased perfusion of the anterior cingulate gyrus in OCD patients compared with controls has been found by two groups using ^{99m}Tc-HMPAO SPET[40,120], whereas a third reported increased rCBF in orbitofrontal and parietal cortices and decreased rCBF in the basal ganglia[38]. The later finding is in agreement with clinical studies showing a high incidence of obsessions and compulsions in neurological disorders supposed to affect basal ganglia regions, such as Tourette's syndrome and Sydenham's chorea.

The effects of treatment on rCBF abnormalities in OCD have also been investigated. Preliminary data from a ^{99m}Tc-HMPAO study[121] suggested attentuation of the 'hyperfrontal' pattern after 3 to 4 months of treatment with fluoxetine. No effects were found in the basal ganglia, which is in contrast with previous PET findings of glucose metabolism reductions in the right caudate region after 10 weeks of treatment with either fluoxetine or behavioural therapy[122]. Follow-up studies with larger samples are now needed to fully clarify these findings and investigate the fascinating possibility that behavioural interventions may promote long-standing changes in neural functioning.

Thus, the SPET and PET literature to date indicates dysfunction of neural circuits involving frontal and striatal areas in OCD. These findings have supported theories that relate OCD symptoms to a failure of the striatum in its role of filtering sensory and cognitive information and suppressing intrusive adventitious thoughts and sensations; the patterns of frontal hyperactivity would in turn be related to conscious attempts to suppress those thoughts and feelings[123].

Major depression The notion that a neurobiological substrate underlies the symptoms of major depression has been mainly supported by neurochemical and neuroendocrine evidence, suggesting the presence of abnormal monoaminergic neurotransmission in association with the disorder[124,125]. It remains, however, unclear how the neurotransmitter abnormalities in depression reflect on the functional anatomical organization in the brain. Several functional imaging studies using SPET and other techniques have tried to clarify this question, investigating exploratively the presence of regional metabolic dysfunction in association with symptoms of depression.

In a large ^{133}Xe SPET investigation of a heterogeneous group of major depressive subjects[126], hypoperfusion of temporal and inferior frontal areas was found in a subgroup of 20 unmedicated patients. The finding of decreased frontal rCBF is in agreement with other studies in depression using PET[44,127,128] techniques. An equally large ^{99m}Tc-HMPAO SPET study[129] investigated 40 patients with the diagnosis of unipolar major depression and 20 controls at rest. Several cortical and subcortical regions were hypofunctional, most importantly the inferior frontal, temporal and parietal regions of interest. Moreover, a negative correlation was found between severity of depressive symptoms as defined in the Hamilton scale and rCBF in anterior regions, a relationship described in previous PET[127] and ^{133}Xe inhalation rCBF studies[130].

Disturbances of lateralized function in depression have also been reported. In a case–control ^{123}I-IMP SPET investigation of 32 depressive patients with endogenous features[131], the left hemisphere was found to be, as a whole, significantly less perfused than the right hemisphere. Similar finding were subsequently reported in a ^{133}Xe SPET study of 38 major depressive patients and 16 healthy controls[132]. These results are in agreement with studies investigating emotional disturbances in brain-lesioned patients, which have suggested an association between left-sided lesions and depression[132].

The characterization of functional patterns in elderly patients with depression has also raised interest, mainly for its potential in differentiating the cognitive deficits of dementia from those associated with depressive syndromes. A recent ^{99m}Tc-HMPAO SPET study compared the resting rCBF patterns of 20 old age depressed patients with 20 AD patients and 30 matched normal subjects[104]. Frontal hypofunction was found, as expected, in the depressive group compared with healthy controls. However, the posterior rCBF patterns were remarkably preserved in the depressive group in comparison with the AD group, suggesting that SPET may be of use in the differentiation of the two conditions.

The only ^{99m}Tc-HMPAO SPET activation study in this area, to date, measured rCBF in a small sample of major depressive bipolar patients and depressed schizophrenics during a somatosensory task[68]. Both groups were 'hypofrontal' in comparison with normal volunteers studied at rest, but in different ways; whereas the left dorsolateral prefrontal cortex was more affected in schizophrenics, right inferior portions were the most hypofunctional in the depressed bipolar patients. Different patterns of frontal hypofunction in major depression and schizophrenia have also been reported in a ^{133}Xe inhalation rCBF study during the performance of the WCST[133]. Both studies therefore suggest that distinct mechanisms of frontal dysfunction are involved in the two disorders.

The functional imaging studies reported here suggest decreased blood flow in the left hemisphere and the frontal cortex in association with depression. Agreement is, however, far from complete, with some studies having found no differences between patients and controls[134,135] or even 'hyperfrontality' in unipolar depressives[136].

This controversy is possibly accounted for by the well-known heterogeneity of depressive disorders. Considerable amounts of genetic and pharmacological research suggest biological differences between unipolar and bipolar depression[136]. Moreover, the clinical presentation of the depressive syndrome itself is highly variable, and different symptoms of depression may have specific underlying patterns of brain function. The latter possibility has been recently addressed in an rCBF PET study[45]. In a sample of 40 major depressives, specific blood flow abnormalities were found in association with specific subsyndromes of depression. Psychomotor retardation and depressed mood were associated with reduced dorsolateral prefrontal cortex rCBF; anxiety correlated positively with posterior cingulate and inferior parietal rCBF bilaterally; and cognitive impairment correlated positively with medial prefrontal cortex rCBF.

Thus, future rCBF studies investigating depression will need to include large, well-characterized samples in order to account for the heterogeneity of the syndrome. The ready availability and inexpensiveness of rCBF SPET techniques make them the most suitable tools for that endeavour.

Substance abuse The potential applications of rCBF techniques on drug abuse research have recently been outlined[137]. Studies on the acute effects of drugs may help to unravel the patterns of functional activity underlying the behavioural changes associated with their use; this can provide insights into the understanding of mechanisms of reinforcement associated with drugs of abuse. Imaging chronic drug users, on the other hand, is likely to primarily map the foci of brain damage associated with continued drug use, and help to identify regions that may be particularly vulnerable; functional patterns underlying psychiatric syndromes associated with chronic drug use can also be identified.

Most of the earlier studies have employed PET techniques. A few SPET studies have now also been reported, especially on cocaine and alcohol abuse.

Cocaine Previous PET studies have detected global decreases in glucose utilization after *acute* intravenous administration of cocaine to normal volunteers[138]. A recent ^{99m}Tc-HMPAO SPET study also showed decreased frontal and basal ganglia rCBF after acute intravenous administration of cocaine to abstinent chronic drug abusers[139]; these rCBF reductions were correlated with self-report measures of euphoriant effects. The addictive and reinforcement behaviours associated with cocaine use are thought to be related to the drug's effects on dopaminergic function. The SPET findings above suggest that abnormal dopaminergic transmission specifically in frontal and striatal regions may be related to the euphoriant and reinforcement effects associated with cocaine use[139]. Recent support for such a relationship has also come from a PET dual imaging study in cocaine abusers[140] measuring both glucose metabolism and D2 receptor density with the [^{18}F]N-methylspiroperidol method. This study showed a clear association between decreased glucose metabolism in frontal areas and decreased striatal dopamine D2 receptor availability.

A recent PET study also demonstrated decreased relative prefrontal rCBF in *chronic*, neurologically intact cocaine users in the early stages of abstinence[141]. Preliminary follow-up data suggest that this pattern persists after 3–4 months of detoxification[142], and correlates in severity with the amount and duration of cocaine use. SPET studies using ^{99m}Tc-HMPAO[143,144] also found frontal as well as other cortical and subcortical foci of hypoperfusion in recently abstinent, chronic cocaine users. However, in contrast with the PET findings above, the latter studies showed amelioration of the rCBF defects after one month of abstinence[145]. Longer follow-up studies, taking into account duration and pattern of cocaine use, are now needed to clarify the extent to which drug-related patterns of hypoperfusion are reversible on a long-term basis.

Alcohol A few functional imaging studies have investigated the patterns of cerebral function during *acute* alcoholic intoxication. In moderate quantities (up to 0.5 g/kg), small rCBF increases have been noted[146], maybe related to the disinhibiting effects of alcohol at that dose level. Studies using larger doses (0.8 to 1.0 g/kg) have, on the other hand, shown both rCBF and glucose metabolism reductions[147–149]. Although the rCBF findings above may be related to alcohol-induced changes in neuronal function, they may also reflect, at least in part, the potent vasoactive actions of the drug.

A recent ^{133}Xe SPET study[150] assessed the effects of *chronic* alcohol use in 20 subjects. Focal reductions were found in frontal, occipital and parietal regions, and could not be accounted for only by alcohol-related brain atro-

Table 3. *rCBF SPET studies – clinical applications in psychiatry*

Current applications
Differential diagnosis between dementia and depressive pseudo-dementia
Differential diagnosis between Alzheimer's disease and multi-infarct dementia
Exclusion of organic disease in cases with unusual psychiatric symptomatology
Detection of central nervous system involvement in systemic diseases such as
- Systemic lupus erythematosus
- Chronic fatigue syndrome

and others

Potential applications
Early diagnosis of Alzheimer's disease
Diagnosis of HIV encephalopathy in its early stages
Differential diagnosis between schizophrenia and depression (activation studies)
Prediction of response to treatment and prognosis of psychiatric disorders

phy as assessed with CT scan. This pattern of hypoperfusion is consistent with previous ^{133}Xe rCBF studies[137] as well as PET data[151,152], and may underlie the cognitive deficits associated with alcohol abuse.

A ^{99m}Tc-HMPAO SPET study[109] investigated the resting rCBF patterns of 10 patients suffering from the more circumscribed alcohol-related Korsakoff's psychosis. Trends towards frontal hypoperfusion were found, and correlated with the memory and orientation deficits typically found in the syndrome.

Clinical applications

The abundance of blood flow abnormalities in psychiatric disorders suggest that hopes of major clinical applications for SPET techniques may be fulfilled in the near future. Table 3 gives some of the currently accepted and potential applications for rCBF SPET studies in psychiatry.

Clear clinical applications have already been proposed in the evaluation of dementing disorders. The addition of SPET to clinical criteria increases the diagnostic confidence with which AD cases can be distinguished from normals to almost 100%[153].

Although CT and MRI are the instruments of choice in the distinction between AD and treatable forms of dementia, some studies have suggested a role for SPET, particularly in the distinction of AD from multi-infarct dementia[154]; in contrast to the usual temporo-parietal pattern of hypofunction usually seen in AD, multiple foci of hypoperfusion are typically detected in multi-infarct dementia, involving both cortical and subcortical structures[36]. A role for SPET has also been suggested in the diagnosis of the so-called frontal lobe dementias (such as Pick's disease), in which patterns of frontal hypoperfusion would be more prominent, in distinction to the more posterior deficits seen in AD. Recently, however, frontal rCBF dysfunction has been reported in the early stages of AD[108], suggesting that SPET may not reliably differentiate the two syndromes. Other potential applications of SPET in dementia include the diagnosis of AD in its early stages, where only mild cognitive impairment is seen and structural imaging studies may be inconclusive; activation paradigms may have a role to play in those cases, challenging areas which may only be subtly dysfunctional.

Possible clinical applications of SPET in the clinical diagnosis and management of AIDS have also been proposed. Preliminary reports have suggested that SPET is sensitive enough to detect diffuse hypoperfusion deficits in early stages of the disease[155,156], when mild cognitive deficits or psychotic symptoms are present but the diagnosis of HIV encephalopathy is still uncertain. Attentuation of these perfusion deficits has been shown after zidovudine (AZT) therapy[156]. A very high incidence of multiple perfusion defects has also been described in cases of definite AIDS dementia complex, although these seem to be indistinguishable from findings in non-HIV-positive cocaine polydrug abusers[144].

The low specificity of blood flow patterns in other psychiatric disorders inhibits wider diagnostic application of rCBF SPET studies at present. However, the recent findings of differential blood flow patterns in schizophrenics and major depressives during activation tasks[68,133] suggest that these paradigms may have diagnostic applications in the near future. Moreover, the consistency of other findings, such as the orbitofrontal hyperactivity in unmedicated OCD patients, already warrants further investigation of their possible applications in predicting prognosis and evaluating response to treatment.

Acknowledgement

G F Busatto is sponsored by the Conselho de Desenvolvimento Cientifico e Tecnologico (CNPq), Brazil.

References

(1) Roy CS, Sherrington CS. On the regulation of the blood supply of the brain. *J Physiol Lond* 1890; 11: 85–108.

(2) Kety SS, Schmidt CF. The nitrous oxide method for the quantitative determination of cerebral blood flow in man: theory, procedure and normal values. *J Clin Invest* 1948; 27: 107–19.

(3) Ingvar DH, Schwartz MS. Blood flow patterns induced in the dominant hemisphere by speech and reading. *Brain* 1974; 97: 273–88.

(4) Roland PE, Meyer E, Shibasaki YL, Yamamoto YL, Thompson CJ. Regional cerebral blood flow changes in cortex and basal ganglia during voluntary movements in normal human volunteers. *J Neurophysiol* 1982; 48: 467–80.

(5) Fox PT, Raichle ME. Stimulus rate dependence of regional cerebral blood flow in human striate cortex demonstrated by positron emission tomography. *J Neurophysiol* 1984; 51: 1109–20.
(6) Woods SW, Hegeman IM, Zubal IG et al. Visual stimulation increases technetium-[^{99m}]-HMPAO distribution in human visual cortex. *J Nucl Med* 1991; 32: 210–15.
(7) Raichle ME. Circulatory and metabolic correlates of brain function in normal humans. In: Plum F, ed. *The nervous system: higher functions of the brain.* Bethesda: American Physiological Society; 1987: 643–74.
(8) Sokoloff L. Localization of functional activity in the central nervous system by measurement of glucose utilization with radioactive deoxyglucose. *J Cereb Blood Flow Metab* 1981; 1: 7–36.
(9) Madsen PL. Cerebral blood flow (CBF) and cerebral metabolic rate (CMR) during sleep and wakefulness. *Acta Neurol Scand* 1993; 88 (suppl 148).
(10) Baron JC, Rougemont D, Collard P, Bustany, P, Bousser MG, Comar D. Coupling between cerebral blood flow, oxygen consumption, and glucose utilization: its study with positron emission tomography. In: Reivich M, Alavi, A, eds. *Positron emission tomography.* New York: Alan R. Liss; 1980: 203–18.
(11) Frackowiak RSJ, Lenzi GL, Jones T, Heather JD. Quantitative measurement of regional cerebral blood flow and oxygen metabolism in man using ^{15}O and positron emission tomography: theory, procedure and normal values. *J Comp Ass Tomog* 1980; 4: 727–36.
(12) Ingvar DH, Lassen NA. Regional cerebral blood flow of the cerebral cortex determined by ^{85}krypton. *Acta Physiol Scand* 1963; 54: 325–38.
(13) Hoedt-Rasmussen L, Sveinsdottir E, Lassen NA. Regional cerebral blood flow in man determined by intra-arterial injection of radioactive inert gas. *Circ Res* 1963; 18: 237–47.
(14) Veall N, Mallett BL. The two-compartment model using ^{133}Xe inhalation and external counting. *Acta Neurol Scand* 1965; 14 (suppl): 83–4.
(15) Costa DC. Single photon emission tomography (SPET) with 99Tc^{m}-hexamethylpropyleneamineoxime (HMPAO) in research and clinical practice – a useful tool. *Vasc Med Rev* 1990; 1: 179–201.
(16) Lassen AN, Sveindottir E, Kanno I, Stokely EM, Rommer P. A fast moving, single photon emission tomograph for regional cerebral blood flow studies in man. *J Comp Ass Tomog* 1978; 2: 661–2.
(17) Verhoeff NPLG, Buell U, Costa DC et al. Basic recommendations for brain SPECT. *Nuklearmedizin* 1992; 31: 114–31.
(18) Neirinckx RD, Canning LR, Piper IM et al. Technetium-99m d,l-HM-PAO: a new radiopharmaceutical for SPECT imaging of regional cerebral blood perfusion. *J Nucl Med* 1987; 28: 191–202.
(19) Holman BL, Lee RGL, Hill TC, Lovett RD, Lister-James J. A comparison of two cerebral perfusion tracers. *N*-isopropyl-I-123 *p*-iodoamphetamine and I-123 HIPDM in the human. *J Nucl Med* 1984; 25: 25–30.
(20) Greenberg JH, Kushner M, Rango M et al. Validation studies of iodine-123-iodoamphetamine as a cerebral blood flow tracer using emission tomography. *J Nucl Med* 1990; 31: 1364–9.
(21) Léveillé J, Demonceau G, De Roo M et al. Characterization of

technetium-99m-L,L-ECD for brain perfusion imaging, part 2: biodistribution and brain imaging in humans. *J Nucl Med* 1989; 30: 1902–10.

(22) Royal HD, Hill TC, Holman BL. Clinical brain imaging with iso-propyl-iodoamphetamine and SPECT. *Semin Nucl Med* 1985; 15: 357–76.

(23) Nakano S, Kinoshita K, Jinnouchi S et al. Critical cerebral blood flow thresholds studied by SPECT using xenon-133 and iodine-123 iodoamphetamine. *J Nucl Med* 1989; 30: 337–42.

(24) Ell PJ, Cullum I, Costa DC. Regional cerebral blood flow mapping with a new Tc-99m-labelled compound. *Lancet* 1985; ii: 50–1.

(25) Sharp PF, Smith FW, Gemmell HG et al. Technetium-99m-HM-PAO stereoisomers as potential agents for imaging regional cerebral blood flow. *J Nucl Med* 1986; 27: 171–7.

(26) Inugami A, Kanno I, Uemura K et al. Linearization correction of ^{99m}Tc-labeled hexamethyl-propylene amine oxime (HM-PAO) image in terms of regional CBF distribution; comparison of $^{15}O_2$ inhalation steady-state method measured by positron emission tomography. *J Cereb Blood Flow Metab* 1988; 8 (suppl 1): S52–60.

(27) Heiss WD, Herholz K, Podreka I, Neubauer I, Pietrzyk U. Comparison of [99mTc]HMPAO SPECT with [18F]Fluoromethane PET in cerebrovascular disease. *J Cereb Blood Flow Metab* 1990; 10: 687–97.

(28) Andersen A, Hasselbach SG, Lassen NA, Kristensen K, Paulson OB, Neirinckx RD. Tc-99m-HMPAO d,l imaging of CBF: a comparison with xenon-133 [Abstract]. *J Cereb Blood Flow Metab* 1987; 7 (suppl 1): S559.

(29) Lassen NA, Andersen AR, Friberg L, Paulson OB. The retention of 99mTc-d,l HM-PAO in the human brain after intra-carotid bolus injection: a kinetic analysis. *J Cereb Blood Flow Metab* 1988; 8 (suppl 1): 13–22.

(30) Rubin P, Holm S, Friberg L et al. Altered modulation of prefrontal and subcortical brain activity in newly diagnosed schizophrenia and schizophreniform disorder. A regional cerebral blood flow study. *Arch Gen Psychiat* 1991; 48: 987–95.

(31) Léveillé J, Demonceau G, Walovitch RC. Intrasubject comparison between technetium-99m-ECD and technetium-99m-HMPAO in healthy human subjects. *J Nucl Med* 1992; 33: 480–4.

(32) George MS, Ring HA, Costa DC, Ell PJ, Kouris K, Jarritt P. *Neuroactivation and neuroimaging with SPET.* London: Springer; 1991.

(33) Holm S, Madsen PL, Sperling B, Lassen NA. Visual activation response with Tc-99m ECD (Neurolite): validation of a split-dose method [Abstract]. *J Cereb Blood Flow Metab* 1993; 13 (suppl 1): S335.

(34) Kouris K, Jarritt PH, Costa DC, Ell PJ. Physical assessment of the GE/CGR NEUROCAM and comparison to a single rotating gamma camera. *Eur J Nucl Med* 1992; 19: 236–42.

(35) Jarritt PJ, Kouris K. Instrumentation for SPET. Guidelines and quantification. Presented at the post-congress meeting 'New Trends in Nuclear Neurology' of the annual European Congress of Nuclear Medicine; August 28, 1992; Funchal, Madeira.

(36) Holman BL, Devous MD. Functional brain SPECT: the emergence of a powerful clinical method. *J Nucl Med* 1992; 33: 1888–904.

(37) Costa DC, Ell PJ, Burns A, Philpot M, Levy R. CBF tomograms with [99mTc-HM-PAO] in patients with dementia (Alzheimer type and HIV) and Parkinson's disease. Initial results. *J Cereb Blood Flow Metab* 1988; 8 (suppl 1): S109–15.
(38) Rubin RT, Villanueva-Meyer J, Ananth J, Trajmar PG, Mena I. Regional xenon 133 cerebral blood flow and cerebral technetium 99m HMPAO uptake in unmedicated patients with obsessive–compulsive disorder and matched normal control subjects. *Arch Gen Psychiat* 1992; 49: 695–702.
(39) Shedlack KJ, Hunter R, Wyper D, McLuskie R, Fink G, Goodwin GM. The pattern of cerebral activity underlying verbal fluency shown by split-dose single photon emission tomography (SPET or SPECT) in normal volunteers. *Psychol Med* 1991; 21: 687–96.
(40) Machlin SR, Harris GJ, Pearson GD, Hoehn-Saric R, Jeffery P, Camargo EE. Elevated medial–frontal cerebral blood flow in obsessive–compulsive patients: a SPECT study. *Am J Psychiat* 1991; 148: 1240–2.
(41) Mazziotta JC, Valentino D, Pelizzari CA, Chen GT, Bookstein F. Structure–function correlation of the living human brain with MRI and PET: a means of anatomical and functional localization. *Clin Neuropharmacol* 1990; 13 (suppl 2): 460–1.
(42) Harris GJ, Pearlson GD. MRI-guided region of interest placement on emission computed tomograms. *Psychiat Res: Neuroimaging* 1993; 50: 57–63.
(43) Friston KJ, Frith CD, Liddle PF, Frackowiak RSJ. Comparing functional (PET) images: the assessment of significant change. *J Cereb Blood Flow Metab* 1991; 11: 690–9.
(44) Bench CJ, Friston KJ, Brown RG, Scott LC, Frackowiak RSJ, Dolan RJ. The anatomy of melancholia – focal abnormalities of cerebral blood flow in major depression. *Psychol Med* 1992; 22: 607–15.
(45) Bench CJ, Friston KJ, Brown RG, Frackowiak RSJ, Dolan RJ. Regional cerebral blood flow in depression measured by positron emission tomography: the relationship with clinical dimensions. *Psychol Med* 1993; 23: 579–90.
(46) Haxby JV, Horwitz B, Maisog JM et al. Frontal and temporal participation in long-term recognition memory for faces: a PET–rCBF activation study [Abstract]. *J Cereb Blood Flow Metab* 1993; 13 (suppl 1): S499.
(47) Rauch SL, Jenike MA, Alpert NM, Baer L, Brieter HCR, Fischman AJ. Measurement of rCBF during symptom provocation in obsessive–compulsive disorder [Abstract]. *J Cereb Blood Flow Metab* 1993; 13 (suppl 1): S526.
(48) Gur RE, Gur RC, Resnick SM, Skolnick BE, Alavi A, Reivich M. The effect of anxiety on cortical blood flow and metabolism. *J Cereb Blood Flow Metab* 1987; 7: 173–7.
(49) Mountz JM, Modell JG, Wilson M et al. Positron emission tomographic evaluation of cerebral blood flow during state anxiety in simple phobia. *Arch Gen Psychiat* 1989; 46: 501–4.
(50) Zohar J, Insel TR, Berman KF, Foa EB, Hill JL, Weinberger DR. Anxiety

and cerebral blood flow during behavioural challenge. Dissociation of central from peripheral and subjective measures. *Arch Gen Psychiat* 1989; 46: 505–10.
(51) Reiman EM, Fusselman MJ, Fox PT, Raichle ME. Neuroanatomical correlates of anticipatory anxiety. *Science* 1989; 243: 1071–4.
(52) Drevets WC, Videen T, MacLeod AK, Haller JW, Raichle ME. PET images of blood flow changes during anxiety: correction. *Science* 1992; 256: 1696.
(53) O'Carroll RE, Moffoot APR, Van Beck M et al. The effect of anxiety induction on the regional uptake of 99mTc-exametazime in simple phobia as shown by single photon emission tomography (SPET). *J Aff Dis* 1993; 28: 203–10.
(54) Gur RE, Gur RC, Obrist WD et al. Sex and handedness differences in cerebral blood flow during rest and cognitive activity. *Science* 1982; 217: 659–61.
(55) Warkentin S, Rodriguez G, Risberg J, Rosaldini G. Sex differences in regional cerebral blood flow (rCBF) [Abstract]. *J Cereb Blood Flow Metab* 1987; 7 (suppl 1): S228.
(56) Gur RC, Gur RE, Obrist WD, Skolnick BE, Reivich M. Age and regional cerebral blood flow at rest and during cognitive activity. *Arch Gen Psychiat* 1987; 44: 617–21.
(57) Marchal G, Rioux P, Petit-Taboue MC et al. Regional cerebral oxygen consumpton, blood flow, and blood volume in healthy human aging. *Arch Neurol* 1992; 49: 1013–20.
(58) Duara R, Gross-Glenn K, Barker WW et al. Behavioral activation and the variability of cerebral glucose metabolic measurements. *J Cereb Blood Flow Metab* 1987; 7: 266–71.
(59) Weinberger DR, Berman KF, Zec RF. Physiologic dysfunction of dorsolateral prefrontal cortex in schizophrenia I. Regional cerebral blood flow evidence. *Arch Gen Psychiat* 1986; 43: 114–24.
(60) Berman KF. Cortical 'stress tests' in schizophrenia: regional cerebral blood flow studies. *Biol Psychiat* 1987; 22: 1304–26.
(61) Buchsbaum MS, DeLisi LE, Holcomb HH et al. Anteroposterior gradients in cerebral glucose use in schizophrenia and affective disorders. *Arch Gen Psychiat* 1984; 41: 1159–66.
(62) Lewis SW, Ford RA, Syed GM, Reveley AM, Toone BK. A controlled study of 99mTc-HMPAO single-photon emission imaging in chronic schizophrenia. *Psychol Med* 1992; 22: 27–35.
(63) Holm S, Madsen PL, Rubin P, Sperling B, Friberg L, Lassen NA. Tc-99m HMPAO activation studies: validation of the split-dose, image subtraction approach [Abstract]. *J Cereb Blood Flow Metab* 1991; 11 (suppl 2): S766.
(64) Busatto GF, Costa DC, Ell PJ, Pilowsky LS, David AS, Kerwin RW. Regional cerebral blood flow (rCBF) in schizophrenia during verbal memory activation: a ^{99m}TcHMPAO single photon emission tomography (SPET) study. *Psychol Med* 1994; 24: 463–72.
(65) Kawasaki Y, Maeda Y, Suzuki M et al. SPECT analysis of regional cerebral

blood flow changes in patients with schizophrenia during the Wisconsin Card Sorting Test. *Schizophrenia Res* 1993; 10: 109–16.
(66) Moffoot A, O'Carroll RE, Murray C, Dougall N, Ebmeyer K, Goodwin GM. Clonidine infusion increases uptake of ^{99M}Tc-exametazime in anterior cingulate cortex in Korsakoff's psychosis. *Psychol Med* 1993; 24: 53–62.
(67) Riddle W, O'Carroll RE, Dougall NJ et al. A single photon emission computerised tomography study of regional brain function underlying verbal memory in patients with Alzheimer-type dementia. *Br J Psychiat* 1993; 163: 166–72.
(68) Ebert D, Feistel H, Barocka A, Kaschka W, Mokrusch T. A test–retest study of cerebral blood flow during somatosensory stimulation in depressed patients with schizophrenia and major depression. *Eur Arch Clin Neurosci* 1992; 242: 250–4.
(69) Brown R, Colter N, Corsellis JAN et al. Post-mortem evidence of structural brain changes in schizophrenia: differences in brain weight, temporal horn area and parahippocampal gyrus compared with affective disorder. *Arch Gen Psychiat* 1986; 43: 36–42.
(70) Bogerts B, Meertz E, Schonfeldt-Bausch R. Basal ganglia and limbic system pathology in schizophrenia: a morphometric study of brain volume and shrinkage. *Arch Gen Psychiat* 1985; 42: 784–91.
(71) Falkai P, Bogerts B. Cell loss in the hippocampus of schizophrenics. *Eur Arch Psychiat Neurol Sci* 1986; 236: 154–61.
(72) Benes F, McSparren J, Bird ED. Deficits in small interneurons in prefrontal and cingulate cortices of schizophrenic and schizo-affective patients. *Arch Gen Psychiat* 1991; 48: 996–1001.
(73) Johnstone EC, Crow TJ, Frith CD, Husband J, Kreel L. Cerebral ventricular size and cognitive impairment in chronic schizophrenia. *Lancet* 1976; ii: 924–6.
(74) Suddath RI, Christison GW, Fuller-Torrey E, Casanova MF, Weinberger DR. Anatomical abnormalities in the brains of monozygotic twins discordant for schizophrenia. *N Engl J Med* 1990; 322: 789–94.
(75) Bogerts B, Ashtari M, Degreef G, Alvir JMJ, Bilder RM, Lieberman JA. Reduced temporal limbic structure volumes on magnetic resonance images in first episode schizophrenia. *Psychiat Res: Neuroimaging* 1990; 35: 1–13.
(76) Shenton ME, Kikinis R, Jolesz FA et al. Abnormalities of the left temporal lobe and thought disorder in schizophrenia. A quantitative magnetic resonance imaging study. *N Engl J Med* 1992; 327: 604–12.
(77) Ingvar DH, Franzén G. Abnormalities of cerebral blood distribution in patients with chronic schizophrenia. *Acta Psychiat Scand* 1974; 50: 425–62.
(78) Matthew RJ, Wilson WH, Tant SR, Robinson L, Prakash R. Abnormal resting regional cerebral blood flow patterns and their correlates in schizophrenia. *Arch Gen Psychiat* 1988; 45: 542–9.
(79) Wilson WH, Matthew RJ. Asymmetry of rCBF in schizophrenia: relationship to AP-gradient and duration of illness. *Biol Psychiat* 1993; 33: 806–14.

(80) Buchsbaum MS, Ingvar DH, Kessler R et al. Cerebral glucography with positron emission tomography. *Arch Gen Psychiat* 1982; 39: 251–9.
(81) Farkas T, Wolf AP, Jaeger J, Brodie JD, Christman DR, Fowler JS. Regional brain glucose metabolism in chronic schizophrenia. *Arch Gen Psychiat* 1984; 41: 293–300.
(82) Wolkin A, Jaeger J, Jonathan DB et al. Persistence of cerebral metabolic abnormalities in chronic schizophrenia as determined by positron emission tomography. *Am J Psychiat* 1985; 142: 564–571.
(83) Volkow ND, Brodie JD, Wolf AP et al. Brain organization in schizophrenia. *J Cereb Blood Flow Metab* 1986; 6: 441–6.
(84) Buchsbaum MS, Nuechterlein KH, Haier RJ et al. Glucose metabolic rate in normals and schizophrenics during the Continuous Performance Test assessed by positron emission tomography. *Br J Psychiat* 1990; 156: 216–27.
(85) Vita A, Cazullo CL, Invernizzi G. Cerebral SPECT in drug free schizophrenic patients [Abstract]. *Schizophrenia Res* 1990; 3: 24.
(86) Paulman RG, Devous MD, Gregory RR et al. Hypofrontality and cognitive impairment in schizophrenia: dynamic Single Photon Emission Tomography and neuropsychological assessment of schizophrenic brain function. *Biol Psychiat* 1990; 27: 377–99.
(87) Siegel BV, Buchsbaum MS, Bunney WE et al. Cortical–striatal–thalamic circuits and brain glucose metabolic activity in 70 unmedicated male schizophrenic patients. *Am J Psychiat* 1993; 150: 1325–36.
(88) Early TS, Reiman SM, Raichle ME, Spitznagel EL. Left globus pallidus abnormality in never-medicated patients with schizophrenia. *Proc Natl Acad Sci USA* 1987; 84: 561–3.
(89) Buchsbaum MS, Wu J, DeLisi LE et al. Positron emission tomography studies of basal ganglia and somatosensory cortex neuroleptic drug effects: differences between normal controls and schizophrenic patients. *Biol Psychiat* 1987; 22: 479–94.
(90) Buchsbaum MS. The frontal lobes, basal ganglia, and temporal lobes as sites for schizophrenia. *Schizophrenia Bull* 1990; 16: 379–89.
(91) DeLisi L, Buchsbaum MS, Holcomb HH et al. Increased temporal lobe glucose use in chronic schizophrenic patients. *Biol Psychiat* 1989; 25: 835–51.
(92) Friston KJ, Liddle PF, Frith CD, Hirsch SR, Frackowiak RSJ. The medial temporal region in schizophrenia. A PET study. *Brain* 1992; 115: 367–82.
(93) Tamminga CA, Thaker GK, Buchanan R et al. Limbic system abnormalities identified in schizophrenia using positron emission tomography with fluorodeoxyglucose and neocortical alterations with deficit syndrome. *Arch Gen Psychiat* 1992; 49: 522–30.
(94) Sheppard G, Manchanda R, Gruzelier J et al. 15-O Positron emission tomography scanning in predominantly never-treated acute schizophrenia patients. *Lancet* 1983; ii: 1448–52.
(95) Gur RE, Resnick SF, Alavi A et al. Regional brain function in schizophrenia. I. A positron emission tomography study. *Arch Gen Psychiat* 1987; 44: 119–25.

(96) Szetchman H, Nahmias C, Garnett S et al. Effect of neuroleptics on altered cerebral glucose metabolism in schizophrenia. *Arch Gen Psychiat* 1988; 45: 523–32.
(97) Ebmeyer KP, Blackwood DHR, Murray C et al. Single-photon emission computed tomography with 99mTc-exametazime in unmedicated schizophrenic patients. *Biol Psychiat* 1993; 33: 487–95.
(98) Liddle PF, Friston KJ, Frith CD, Hirsch SR, Jones T, Frackowiak RSJ. Patterns of cerebral blood flow in schizophrenia. *Br J Psychiat* 1991; 160: 179–86.
(99) McGuire PK, Shah GMS, Murray RM. Increased blood flow in Broca's area during auditory hallucinations in schizophrenia. *Lancet* 1993; ii: 703–6.
(100) David AS. The neuropsychological origin of auditory hallucinations. In: David AS, Cutting J, eds. *Neuropsychology of schizophrenia.* Hove, Sussex: Laurence Erlbaum Associates Ltd; 1993: 269–313.
(101) Neary D, Snowden J, Shields R et al. Single photon emission tomography using 99mTc-HMPAO in the investigation of dementia. *J Neurol, Neurosurg Psychiat* 1987; 50: 1101–9.
(102) Burns A, Philpot MP, Costa DC, Ell PJ, Levy R. The investigation of Alzheimer's disease with single photon emission tomography. *J Neurol, Neurosurg Psychiat* 1989; 52: 248–53.
(103) Montaldi D, Brooks DN, McColl JH, Wyper DJ, Patterson J, Barron E, McCulloch J. Measurements of regional cerebral blood flow and cognitive performance in Alzheimer's disease. *J Neurol, Neurosurg Psychiat* 1990; 53: 33–8.
(104) Curran SM, Murray CM, Van Beck M et al. A single photon emission computerised tomography study of regional brain function in elderly patients with major depression and with Alzheimer-type dementia. *Br J Psychiat* 1993; 163: 155–65.
(105) Frackowiak RSJ, Pozzilli C, Legg NJ et al. Regional cerebral oxygen supply and utilization in dementia. A clinical and physiological study with oxygen-15 and positron tomography. *Brain* 1981; 104: 753–78.
(106) Duara R, Grady C, Haxby JV et al. Positron emission tomography in Alzheimer's disease. *Neurology* 1986; 36: 879–87.
(107) Grady CL, Haxby JV, Schlageter NL, Berg G, Rapoport SI. Stability of metabolic and neuropsychological asymmetries in dementia of the Alzheimer type. *Neurology* 186; 36: 1390–2.
(108) O'Brien JT, Eagger S, Syed GMS, Sahakian BJ, Levy R. A study of regional cerebral blood flow and cognitive performance in Alzheimer's disease. *J Neurol, Neurosurg Psychiat* 1993; 55: 1182–7.
(109) Hunter R, McLuskie R, Wyper DJ et al. The pattern of function-related cerebral blood flow investigated by single photon emission tomography with 99mTc-HMPAO in patients with presenile Alzheimer's disease and Korsakoff's psychosis. *Psychol Med* 1989; 19: 847–55.
(110) Deutsch G, Halsey Jr JH, Brooks KW, Rossor MN. Exaggerated cortical blood flow reactivity in early Alzheimer's disease during task performance. *J Cereb Blood Flow Metab* 1993; 13 (suppl 1): S4.
(111) Duara R, Barker WW, Chang J, Yoshii F, Loewenstein DA, Pascal S.

Viability of neocortical function shown in behavioral activation state PET studies in Alzheimer disease. *J Cereb Blood Flow Metab* 1992; 12: 927–34.

(112) Blass JP. Pathophysiology of the Alzheimer's syndrome. *Neurology* 1993; 43 (suppl 4): S25–38.

(113) Geaney PD, Soper N, Shepstone BJ, Cowen PJ. Effect of central cholinergic stimulation on regional cerebral blood flow in Alzeimer's disease. *Lancet* 1990; i: 1484–7.

(114) Hunter R, Wyper DJ, Patterson J, Hansen MT, Goodwin GM. Cerebral pharmacodynamics of physostigmine in Alzheimer's disease investigated using single-photon computerised tomography. *Br J Psychiat* 1991; 158: 351–7.

(115) Ebmeyer KP, Hunter R, Curran SM et al. Effects of a single dose of the acetylcholinesterase inhibitor velnacrine on recognition memory and regional cerebral blood flow in Alzheimer's disease. *Psychopharmacology* 1992; 108: 103–9.

(116) Terry RD, Masliah E, Salmon DP et al. Physical basis of cognitive alterations in Alzheimer's disease: synapse loss is the major correlate of cognitive impairment. *Ann Neurol* 1991; 30: 572–80.

(117) Baxter LR, Schwartz JM, Mazziotta JC et al. Cerebral glucose metabolic rates in nondepressed patients with obsessive–compulsive disorder. *Am J Psychiat* 1988; 145: 1560–3.

(118) Nordahl TE, Benkelfat C, Semple WE, Gross M, King AC, Cohen RM. Cerebral glucose metabolic rates in obsessive–compulsive disorder. *Neuropsychopharmacology* 1989; 2: 23–8.

(119) Swedo SE, Shapiro MB, Grady CL et al. Cerebral glucose metabolism in childhood-onset obsessive–compulsive disorder. *Arch Gen Psychiat* 1989; 46: 518–23.

(120) Goodman WK, McDougle CJ, Price LH et al. SPECT imaging of obsessive–compulsive disorder with Tc99m, d,l-HMPAO [Abstract]. *J Nucl Med* 1990; 31: 750.

(121) Hoehn-Saric R, Pearlson GD, Harris GJ, Machlin SR, Camargo EE. Effects of fluoxetine on regional cerebral blood flow in obsessive–compulsive patients. *Am J Psychiat* 1991; 148: 1243–5.

(122) Baxter LR, Schwartz JM, Bergman KS et al. Caudate glucose metabolic rate changes with both drug and behavior therapy for obsessive–compulsive disorder. *Arch Gen Psychiat* 1992; 49: 681–9.

(123) Baxter LR. Brain imaging as a tool in establishing a theory of brain pathology in obsessive–compulsive disorder. *J Clin Psychiat* 1990; 51 (suppl 2): 22–5.

(124) Heninger GR, Charney DS. Mechanism of action of antidepresant treatments: implications for the etiology and treatment of depressive disorders. In: Meltzer HY, ed. *Psychopharmacology: the third generation of progress*. New York: Raven Press; 1987: 535–44.

(125) Meltzer HY, Lowy MT. The serotonin hypothesis of depression. In: Meltzer HY, ed. *Psychopharmacology: the third generation of progress*. New York: Raven Press; 1987: 513–26.

(126) Devous MD, Guillion C, Granneman B, Rush AJ. Regional cerebral blood flow alterations in unipolar depression [Abstract]. *J Nucl Med* 1989; 32: 951–2.
(127) Buchsbaum MS, Wu J, DeLisi LE et al. Frontal cortex and basal ganglia metabolic rates assessed by positron emission tomography with [^{18}F]2-deoxyglucose in affective illness. *J Aff Dis* 1986; 10: 137–52.
(128) Baxter LR, Schwartz JM, Phelps ME et al. Reduction of prefrontal cortex metabolism common to three types of depression. *Arch Gen Psychiat* 1989; 46: 243–50.
(129) Austin MP, Dougall N, Ross M et al. Single photon emission tomography with 99mTc-exametazime in major depression and the pattern of brain activity underlying the psychotic/neurotic continuum. *J Aff Dis* 1992; 26: 31–44.
(130) Matthew RJ, Meyer JS, Francis DJ, Semchuk KM, Mortel K, Cleghorn JI. Cerebral blood flow in depression. *Am J Psychiat* 1980; 137: 1449–50.
(131) Kanaya T, Yonekawa M. Regional cerebral blood flow in depression. *Jpn J Psychiat Neurol* 1990; 44: 571–6.
(132) Delvenne V, Delecluse F, Hubain PP, Schoutens A, De Maertelaer V, Mendlewicz J. Regional cerebral blood flow in patients with affective disorders. *Br J Psychiat* 1990; 157: 359–65.
(133) Berman KF, Doran AR, Pickar D, Weinberger DR. Is the mechanism of prefrontal hypofunction in depression the same as in schizophrenia? Regional cerebral blood flow during cognitive activation. *Br J Psychiat* 1993; 162: 183–92.
(134) Silfverskiold P, Risberg J. Regional cerebral blood flow in depression and mania. *Arch Gen Psychiat* 1989; 46: 253–9.
(135) Maes M, Dierckx R, Meltzer HY et al. Regional cerebral blood flow in unipolar depression measured with tc-99m-HMPAO single photon emission tomography: negative findings. *Psychiat Res; Neuroimaging* 1993; 50: 89–92.
(136) Drevets WC, Videen TO, Price JL, Preskorn SH, Carmichael ST, Raichle ME. A functional anatomical study of unipolar depression. *J Neurosci* 1992; 12: 3628–41.
(137) Matthew RJ, Wilson WH. Substance abuse and cerebral blood flow. *Am J Psychiat* 148: 292–305.
(138) London ED, Cascella G, Wong DF et al. Cocaine-induced reduction of glucose utilization in human brain. *Arch Gen Psychiat* 1990; 47: 567–74.
(139) Pearlson GD, Jeffery PJ, Harris GJ, Ross CA, Fischman MW, Camargo EE. Correlation of acute cocaine-induced changes in local cerebral blood flow with subjective effects. *Am J Psychiat* 1993; 150: 495–7.
(140) Volkow ND, Fowler JS, Wang GJ et al. Decreased dopamine D2 availability is associated with reduced frontal metabolism in cocaine abusers. *Synapse* 1993; 14: 169–77.
(141) Volkow ND, Mullani N, Gould KL, Adler S, Krajewski K. Cerebral blood flow in chronic cocaine users: a study with PET. *Br J Psychiat* 1988; 148: 621–6.
(142) Volkow ND, Hitzemann R, Wang GJ, Fowler JS, Wolf AP, Dewey SL. Long-term frontal brain metabolic changes in cocaine abusers. *Synapse* 1992; 11: 184–90.

(143) Holman BL, Carvalho PA, Mendelson J et al. Brain perfusion is abnormal in cocaine-dependent polydrug users: a study using technetium-99m-HMPAO and ASPECT. *J Nucl Med* 1991; 32: 1206–10.
(144) Holman BL, Garada B, Johnson KA et al. A comparison of brain perfusion SPECT in cocaine abuse and AIDS dementia complex [Abstract]. *J Nucl Med* 1992; 33: 887.
(145) Holman BL, Mendelson J, Garada B, Teoh SK, Hallgring E, Johnson KA. Regional cerebral blood flow improves with treatment in chronic cocaine polydrug users [Abstract]. *J Nucl Med* 1992; 33: 887.
(146) Matthew RJ, Wilson WH. Regional cerebral blood flow changes associated with ethanol intoxication. *Stroke* 1986; 17: 1156–9.
(147) Volkow ND, Mullani N, Gould KL et al. Effects of acute alcohol intoxication on cerebral blood flow measured with PET. *Psychiat Res* 1988; 24: 201–9.
(148) de Wit H, Metz J, Wagner N, Cooper M. Behavioral and subjective effects of ethanol: relationship to cerebral metabolism using PET. *Alcoholism: Clin Exp Res* 1990; 14: 482–9.
(149) Volkow ND, Hitzemann R, Wolf AP et al. Acute effects of ethanol on regional brain glucose metabolism and transport. *Psychiat Res: Neuroimaging* 1990; 35: 39–48.
(150) Melgaard B, Henriksen L, Ahlgren P, Danielsen UT, Sorensen H, Paulson OB. Regional cerebral blood flow in chronic alcoholics measured by single photon emission computerized tomography. *Acta Neurol Scand* 1990; 82: 87–93.
(151) Wik G, Borg S, Sjogren I et al. PET determination of regional cerebral glucose metabolism in alcohol-dependent men and healthy controls using ^{11}C-glucose. *Acta Psychiat Scand* 1988; 78: 234–41.
(152) Volkow ND, Hitzemann R, Wang GJ et al. Decreased brain metabolism in neurologically intact healthy alcoholics. *Am J Psychiat* 1992; 14: 1016–22.
(153) Dewan MJ, Gupta S. Toward a definite diagnosis of Alzheimer's disease. *Compr Psychiat* 1992; 33: 282–90.
(154) Jagust WJ, Budinger TF, Reed BR. The diagnosis of dementia with single photon emission tomography. *Arch Neurol* 1987; 44: 258–62.
(155) Schielke E, Tatsch K, Pfister HW et al. Reduced cerebral blood flow in early stages of human immunodeficiency virus infection. *Arch Neurol* 1990; 47: 1342–5.
(156) Masdeu JC, Yudd A, Van Hertuum RL et al. Single-photon emission computed tomography in human immunodeficiency virus encephalopathy: a preliminary report. *J Nucl Med* 1991; 32: 1471–5.

Neuroreceptor imaging with PET and SPET: research and clinical applications

G F BUSATTO and L S PILOWSKY

Introduction

In 1878, Langley postulated the existence of 'receptive substances' involved in the response to pharmacological agents in tissue[1]. These 'substances' are nowadays known as *receptors*, and are widely accepted to be responsible for mediating the action of both endogenous transmitters and exogenous pharmacological agents[2].

With a number of technological advances throughout this century, it has been possible biochemically to characterize the structure of a variety of specific transmitters and their receptors in the brain as well as study their interactions. Neuroreceptors consist of large protein or glycoprotein molecules located on membrane surfaces[3]. Specific neurotransmitters and drugs are recognized by, and bind to, these structures, inducing an alteration in their spatial configuration. This, in turn, activates second messenger systems inside the cell, which effectuate the physiological response of the transmitter or drug[2].

Using radioactive-labelled ligands and autoradiographic techniques, it is possible to visualize the distribution of several kinds of neuroreceptors in vitro and ex vivo[3,4]. The same principles have now been applied to allow the visualization and measurement of neuroreceptor function in vivo using positron emission tomography (PET) and single photon emission tomography (SPET)[5]. This development provides a unique means to investigate neurochemical abnormalities in psychiatric and neurological conditions as well as to study the mechanism of action of psychotropic drugs.

This chapter will briefly review the basic principles involved in PET and SPET neuroreceptor imaging. It will also attempt to summarize the most relevant literature on some psychiatric and neurological disorders, relating

All correspondence to: Dr G F Busatto, Section of Clinical Neuropharmacology, Department of Psychological Medicine, Institute of Psychiatry, De Crespigny Park, Denmark Hill, London SE5 8AF, UK.

Cambridge Medical Reviews: Neurobiology and Psychiatry Volume 3

imaging findings to the currently accepted pathophysiological theories for those conditions.

PET and SPET receptor imaging: the basics

The general principles involved in PET and SPET imaging have been recently reviewed[5,6], and outlined in the previous chapter of the volume. In this chapter we focus on the application of those principles to the field of neuroreceptor imaging.

Radioligands

These are molecules labelled with either a positron- or photon-emitting isotope, which selectively bind to specific neuroreceptor sites. Ligands which are receptor antagonists are usually preferred, since they tend to have higher affinity for receptors in comparison with agonists and are less likely to produce receptor–drug responses that might interfere with binding estimations[7].

The required properties of radiotracers for neuroreceptor imaging have been described[2,7] and are summarized in Table 1. In essence, a radioligand

Table 1. *Characteristics of an ideal radioligand for neuroreceptor imaging*

- High selectivity and affinity for the targeted receptor
- Adequate lipophilicity to allow easy and rapid crossing of the blood–brain barrier
- Metabolic stability, with low accumulation of active metabolites
- Rapid clearance from sites of non-specific binding
- Rapid elimination from the blood pool
- Absence of clinical effects at receptor saturating doses
- Easy and economically viable synthesis process

should be selective in its receptor binding profile, get quickly to the brain and remain metabolically stable at the site of binding for long enough to allow the acquisition of reliable information on receptor estimates[8].

Radioligands specific for several neurotransmitter systems have been synthesized and evaluated for use with PET and SPET[9]. Those which have been more extensively applied to the investigation of neuropsychiatric conditions are listed in Table 2.

Data acquisition and analysis

Dynamic imaging protocols are currently preferred to obtain PET and SPET receptor binding data[7]. These involve the acquisition of sequential images of the same regions over time after radioligand administration. The region-of-interest approach, traditionally used in PET and SPET studies of

Table 2. *Neuroreceptor radioligands frequently used in neuropsychiatry research*

Receptor system	Receptor subtype	Imaging technique	Radioligand
Dopaminergic	D_2	PET	^{11}C-raclopride
		PET	^{11}C or ^{18}F-N-methylspiperone
		SPET	^{123}I-iodobenzamide (IBZM)
	D_1	PET	^{11}C-SCH23390
Serotonergic	5-HT_2	PET	^{11}C-setoperone
		PET	^{11}C or ^{18}F-N-methylspiperone
Cholinergic	M1 muscarinic	SPET	^{123}I-QNB
Opioid		PET	^{11}C-diprenorphine
GABAergic	$GABA_A$	PET	^{11}C-flumazenil
		SPET	^{123}I-iomazenil

blood flow and glucose metabolism, is also the most commonly employed for analysing receptor images[10–12]. Regions of interest are defined around different brain areas, and regional measures of radioligand uptake obtained.

This process allows the generation of time–activity curves which display the regional brain patterns of radiotracer uptake and washout[13]. Regions with high receptor density show relatively higher radioligand uptake compared with areas of low receptor density, as well as longer time to peak activity and slower tracer washout. In addition, quick radioligand clearance from high receptor density regions is seen if a cold (unlabelled) competitive molecule is administered, whereas in areas with negligible receptor density, displacing agents have no effect[13].

Mathematical models can be applied to dynamic receptor binding data acquired with PET to allow *absolute* quantitation in terms of traditional binding parameters including K_d (equilibrium dissociation constant, related to the *affinity* of the ligand for a specific receptor), and B_{max} (maximal *density* of receptors that specifically bind to the ligand)[2].

Although similar methods have been attempted with SPET[14], problems with attenuation correction, scattering and partial volume effects, make the generation of absolute indices difficult with this technique. However, methods which rely on *relative* measures of specific binding are possible[15], and represent a simple alternative to generate receptor binding estimates comparable with those obtained by absolute quantitation[16]. Semi-

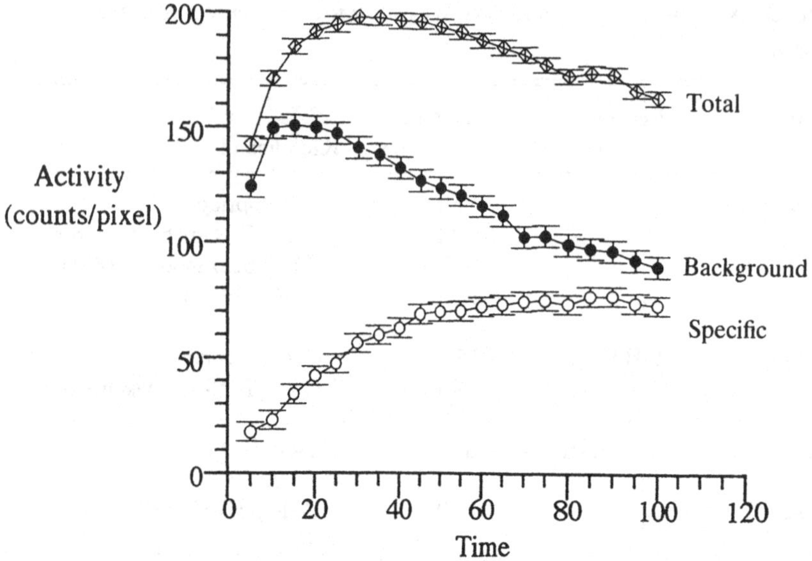

Fig. 1. Mean time–activity curves of ^{123}I-IBZM in healthy controls ($n = 20$). Measures of total activity are given by the radioligand uptake in the striatum (where maximal density of D_2 receptors is seen). Background activity is given by tracer uptake measures in the frontal cortex (which has negligible numbers of D_2 receptors). The data points of the bottom curve represent estimates of 'specific' activity, and are calculated as the difference between striatal and frontal radioligand uptake.

quantitative models assume that, in brain regions rich in a given receptor type, the activity measured represents total radioligand binding (specific binding + non-specific binding + free radioligand), whereas regions presumably free from receptors are used as references for background activity (non-specific binding + free ligand). Relative indices of specific binding are then generated as the ratio or the difference between the measures of total binding and background activity. Fig. 1 displays typical time–activity curves for the dopamine D_2 receptor SPET ligand ^{123}I-iodobenzamide (IBZM) in healthy subjects[8], providing estimates of total activity, background activity and relative measures of 'specific' binding.

Current and potential applications of receptor imaging

Table 3 summarizes the main strategies used in neuroreceptor imaging in vivo studies to date. These have been applied to the evaluation of neuropsychiatric disorders in two major fronts:

- to determine the role of specific receptor systems in the pathophysiology of neuropsychiatric disorders, and

Table 3. *Strategies and applications of receptor imaging studies in neuropsychiatry*

Psychopharmacological studies
- Receptor binding profile of drugs
- Potency of psychotropic drugs – displacement studies
- Dose:receptor occupancy relationship
- Relationship with outcome variables: clinical response/side effects

Studies on the pathophysiology of neuropsychiatric conditions
- Regional abnormalities of receptor density in disease states
- Correlations between receptor binding parameters and clinical variables
- Receptor density abnormalities as a marker of neuronal integrity

- to evaluate interactions of pharmacological agents with receptor systems in order to clarify the mechanism of action of psychotropic drugs and assist the development of alternative treatments.

Schizophrenia

The clinical efficacy of classical antipsychotic drugs is known from in vitro studies to be directly related to their potency to block dopamine D_2 receptors in the brain[17]. This has provided the main basis for the dopamine hypothesis of schizophrenia, which postulates an excessive brain dopaminergic activity in the disorder[18]. Following on from the D_2 blocking action of antipsychotic drugs, a hyperdensity of D_2 receptors might be expected in schizophrenia, as suggested in neurochemical post-mortem studies with medicated patients[19].

In one of the first in vivo studies on the subject, Wong et al[20], using the D_2 receptor tracer ^{11}C-N-methylspiperone (NMSP) and PET, detected in vivo increases in striatal dopamine receptors in medication-free schizophrenics. This could not be replicated by Farde et al[21], who found no elevations of striatal D_2 density in drug-naïve patients using ^{11}C-raclopride PET, or by Martinot et al[22] in a smaller ^{76}Br-bromolisuride PET study. The reasons for those discrepancies have been largely discussed[8], and are likely to relate to methodological differences between studies in terms of behaviour of radioligands and sample selection.

The notion that no overall elevations in striatal D_2 receptor density are present in drug-free schizophrenics has been reinforced in a large ^{123}I-IBZM SPET study by Pilowsky et al[8]. Other abnormalities were, however, detected by those authors, including a failure of patients to show the expected age-related decline in D_2 receptor density, and a relative increase in left D_2 binding in male schizophrenics. This subtle laterality abnormality is in agreement with the left higher than right putaminal D_2 receptor densities in schizophrenics which had been described earlier by Farde et al[21], and adds to a considerable body of literature suggesting the presence of left lateralized brain dysfunction in schizophrenia[23,24].

Although striatal D_2 receptor function has been extensively evaluated in schizophrenia and subtle anomalies found, it is still possible that dopamine receptor abnormalities may be present in extrastriatal regions. Assessment of dopaminergic disturbances in *limbic* regions would be of particular relevance, since schizophrenic symptoms seem to be related more directly to mesolimbic rather than to nigro-striatal dopamine pathways[18,25]. This has not been performed to date owing to insufficient spatial resolution of both PET and SPET imaging devices[26] and limited affinity and sensitivity of radioligands[27]. The latter problem may be overcome with the development of new tracers such as the SPET ligand ^{123}I-epidepride[27].

Pharmacological aspects of the treatment of schizophrenia have also been explored. One ^{11}C-raclopride PET study has found a direct relationship between D_2 blockade and clinical response to typical antipsychotics[28]. This relationship may, however, be valid only for patients who do show some degree of improvement with those drugs, since patients who show no response still present with high levels of D_2 blockade[11]. Moreover, a remarkable antipsychotic response can be obtained with atypical antipsychotics that only weakly block D_2 receptors such as clozapine[15], strongly suggesting that antipsychotic mechanisms alternative to D_2 blockade may be possible.

Finally, the relationship between D_2 blockade and extrapyramidal side effects (EPS) of antipsychotics has been explored, with important implications for understanding the pathophysiology of those symptoms and determining optimal dose ranges for antipsychotic treatment. The latter aim is clear in a recent ^{11}C-raclopride PET study by Farde et al[26]. Investigating patients treated with typical antipsychotics, these authors calculated a threshold of 80% of D_2 receptor occupancy above which EPS are likely to be of clinical significance. Interestingly, however, the relationship between high levels of D_2 blockade and EPS does not seem to be present for all antipsychotics. Using ^{123}I-IBZM SPET, Busatto et al[29] demonstrated a high degree of D_2 blockade in patients treated with the novel antipsychotic risperidone and free from EPS. This finding suggests that additional effects of risperidone (such as its potent blockade of 5-HT_2 receptors) may protect against the appearance of those side effects.

Neurochemical hypotheses for schizophrenia have not been limited to dopaminergic pathways. Post-mortem investigations have suggested that abnormalities of other neurotransmitter systems, such as the glutamatergic and GABAergic, may be involved and even be of primacy over dopaminergic changes[30–32]. It is hoped that the receptor imaging approach will be useful to elucidate those theories in the near future.

Epilepsy

Blood flow and glucose metabolism measurements using PET and SPET have already been applied widely in epilepsy. Their role in the identification of seizure focus in medication-refractory epilepsy is well established, with interictal studies identifying focal hypoactivity in approximately 70% to 75% of cases[5]. The exact pathophysiological mechanisms underlying epileptic seizures are not fully understood. However, a significant role for the inhibitory neurotransmitter gamma-aminobutyric acid (GABA) seems unequivocal[33]. It has therefore been suggested that mapping of the GABA–benzodiazepine (BDZ) receptor complex with PET and SPET may increase the accuracy and sensitivity with which seizure foci can be identified[10].

These advantages have been demonstrated, by comparison of the BDZ antagonist ^{11}C-flumazenil binding with estimates of glucose metabolism with PET. Henry et al[34] investigated 10 patients with medication-resistant partial epilepsy with both techniques. Whereas multifocal abnormalities of glucose metabolism were identified, decreased GABA–BDZ receptor density was found exclusively in medial temporal regions presumed to encompass the seizure focus. Similar findings were also reported by Savic et al[35].

Unfortunately, the results with the more cost-effective SPET technique have not been as encouraging, and no significant advantages of ^{123}I-iomazenil SPET over interictal blood flow imaging have as yet been reported[36,37]. It is, however, indisputable that the binding of ^{123}I-iomazenil is more specific to epileptogenic neurones than that of the blood flow SPET tracer ^{99m}Tc-exametazime (or HMPAO), which presumably binds to neurones as well as glial cells[38]. In addition, when dynamic protocols are used with ^{123}I-iomazenil, additional information may be obtained, such as time to peak radioligand activity and washout rates of specific binding to GABA–BDZ receptors[12].

It is therefore likely that GABA–BDZ receptor imaging will be consolidated not only as a clinically useful tool but also to provide clues to the pathophysiological mechanisms underlying epileptic seizures.

Other potential applications of receptor imaging in partial epilepsy include the prediction of treatment outcome. This has already been hinted in a preliminary ^{11}C-flumazenil PET study by Savic and Thorell[39] showing the severity of focal GABA–BDZ receptor reductions to be directly correlated with the frequency of seizures.

Finally, GABA–BDZ receptor imaging may be useful in the investigation of primary generalized seizures. Using ^{11}C-flumazenil and PET, Savic et al[40] did not identify any focal GABA–BDZ abnormalities in a sample of 10 patients, but found a trend towards low mean cortical receptor density suggestive of diffuse impairments in cortical inhibitory processes in generalized seizures.

Alzheimer's disease (AD)

Although the neuropathological alterations found in AD tend to be widely distributed, a certain degree of selective impairment of specific neurotransmitter pathways can be found. The cholinergic system seems to be specially affected; loss of cholinergic terminals has been described in post-mortem studies[41], and tend to correlate with the severity of dementia[42].

Using the muscarinic-type cholinergic receptor antagonist ^{123}I-QNB and SPET, Weinberger et al[43] studied 12 AD patients in comparison with healthy volunteers, having detected focal receptor reductions in the AD group, mainly in posterior temporal regions. However, it is known that temporal regions tend to be those most affected when regional blood flow is assessed in AD patients[44,45]. It is therefore uncertain if Weinberger et al's findings are due to specific deficits in muscarinic receptors or simply a correlate of regional metabolic abnormalities. Wyper et al[46] looked at this question in a study where eight AD patients had both ^{99m}Tc-HMPAO and ^{123}I-QNB SPET scans. Deficits of ^{123}I-QNB binding not accounted for by blood flow abnormalities were found in only two patients (the most severely demented cases); the remaining patients showed either blood flow deficits only or corresponding deficits with both techniques. These results therefore suggest that ^{123}I-QNB SPET may be of limited use in identifying selective muscarinic receptor deficits in AD.

Other neurochemical abnormalities proposed for the syndrome involve the serotonergic and noradrenergic systems[42]. To date, these have been investigated in only one imaging study by Blin et al[47], who used the 5-HT_2 receptor ligand ^{18}F-setoperone and PET in nine AD patients compared with healthy controls, and identified widespread decreases of cortical binding in the patient group.

Drug abuse

The use of receptor imaging techniques in the field of drug abuse has the potential not only to increase the understanding about mechanisms of action of drugs but also to document the neurochemical consequences of chronic drug administration in dependent subjects.

These avenues have already been explored for *cocaine* use. Volkow et al[48] followed up the uptake and washout of intravenously injected ^{11}C-labelled cocaine with PET. The tracer reached maximal brain accumulation after only 4–8 minutes, concentrating preferentially in the basal ganglia, and was cleared rapidly from the brain (50% of washout after only 20 minutes). In addition, ^{11}C-cocaine was greatly displaced by the dopamine transporter inhibitor nomifensine, but not by other blocking agents. This provides in vivo evidence for the proposed action of cocaine as a potent dopamine reuptake inhibitor.

The chronic consequences of cocaine use on dopaminergic function have also been investigated. Using ^{18}F-NMS and PET, Volkow et al[49] reported decreased striatal D_2 receptor densities in chronic cocaine users soon after drug abstinence. This abnormality has been shown to be present even after 3–4 months of abstinence[50], suggesting that abnormal dopaminergic function in chronic cocaine users is not simply a temporary response to cocaine abstinence, but is probably the reflection of persistent dysfunctional changes of dopaminergic neurotransmission.

The neurochemical consequences of chronic *alcohol* abuse have also been assessed in respect to possible GABA–BDZ receptor abnormalities. In a preliminary ^{11}C-flumazenil PET study, Litton et al[51] quantified the density of GABA receptors in five detoxified chronic alcoholics in comparison with healthy subjects. Although the sample was not large enough to detect differences between the two groups, the values for B_{max} in patients showed a greater variability, with all patients presenting with values outside the range found with controls. These results suggest that GABA–BDZ receptor function may be affected after chronic alcohol abuse, and further research into the area is indicated.

Depression and anxiety

The notion that there is a biological basis to depression has been supported mainly by post-mortem neurochemical and neuroendocrine evidence, suggesting the presence of monoaminergic dysfunction in the syndrome[52,53]. Indeed, virtually all effective antidepressants act by enhancing monoaminergic transmission in the brain[52]. Surprisingly, however, in vivo receptor imaging studies have not yet been reported in depressive syndromes. This may be explained by the relative scarcity of suitable tracers for noradrenaline and serotonin receptors[7].

Abnormalities of several neurotransmitter systems have also been proposed in anxiety disorders, most notably involving GABA, serotonin, noradrenaline and dopamine transmission[54]. The relationship between GABA and anxiety is of special interest, given the action of anxiolytic drugs on the GABA–BDZ receptor complex[55]. In the only receptor imaging study reported to date, Feistel et al[56] found, using ^{123}I-iomazenil SPET, reductions and asymmetries of receptor density in several brain regions of patients presenting with anxiety syndromes, most notably in hippocampal areas. These limbic regions are indeed the most frequently implicated in the genesis of anxiety symptoms[57].

Functional imaging studies have identified regional blood flow and glucose metabolic abnormalities in the frontal lobes of patients suffering from obsessive–compulsive disorder (OCD) with remarkable consistency[58,59]. A primordial role for serotonergic abnormalities has been postulated in OCD[60], making the in vivo mapping of 5-HT_2 receptors in OCD a subject of great interest. The application of dual 5-HT_2 receptor–blood flow/metabolism imaging protocols may be particularly useful to relate the functional anatomical findings to possible serotonergic abnormalities.

Conclusions

The challenges for receptor imaging with PET and SPET have multiplied in the past few years. Molecular genetic studies continually discover new receptor subtypes for many neurotransmitter systems[61,62] with specific properties and possibly specific roles in neuropsychiatric conditions. This increases the urge for the engineering of new radioligands, which must achieve a greater specificity for the described receptor subtypes, retaining the already excellent standards of imaging properties achieved with most of the currently available tracers. These advances will certainly be magnified by the new generation of imaging equipment[6], with improved sensitivity as well as better spatial and temporal resolution.

It is not possible to encompass here the whole range of findings already reported in receptor imaging studies in neuropsychiatry. For instance, the wealth of data available supporting the role of dopamine receptor abnormalities in movement disorders, ably reviewed by Dolan et al[7], has not been discussed.

It is hoped, however, that the enormous potential of these techniques for research and clinical purposes has been made evident, and will stimulate the reader to pursue this area further.

Acknowledgements

G F Busatto is funded by the Conselho Nacional de Desenvolvimento Cientifico e Tecnologico (CNPq), Brazil. L S Pilowsky is a Wellcome Trust Research Training Fellow.

References

(1) Taylor P, Insel PA. Molecular basis of pharmacological selectivity. In: Pratt WB, Taylor P, eds. *Principles of drug action: the basis of pharmacology*. London: Churchill Livingstone; 1990: 1–103.

(2) Sedvall G, Farde L, Persson A, Wiesel F-A. Imaging of neurotransmitter receptors in the living human brain. *Arch Gen Psychiat* 1986; 43: 995–1005.

(3) Maziere B, Maziere M. Where have we got to with neuroreceptor mapping of the human brain? *Eur J Nucl Med* 1990; 16: 817–35.

(4) Sybirska E, al-Tikriti M, Zoghbi SS, Baldwin RM, Johnson EW, Innis RB. SPECT imaging of the benzodiazepine receptor: autoradiographic comparison of receptor density and radioligand distribution. *Synapse* 1992; 12: 119–28.

(5) Holman BL, Devous MD. Functional brain SPECT: the emergence of a powerful clinical method. *J Nucl Med* 1992; 33: 1888–904.

(6) Bailey DL, Zito F, Gilardi M-C, Savi AR, Fazio F, Jones T. Performance

comparison of a state-of-the-art neuro-SPET scanner and a dedicated neuro-PET scanner. *Eur J Nucl Med* 1994; 21: 381–7.
(7) Dolan R, Bench C, Friston K. Positron emission tomography in psychopharmacology. *Int Rev Psychiat* 1990; 2: 427–39.
(8) Pilowsky LS, Costa DC, Ell PJ, Verhoeff NPLG, Murray RM, Kerwin RW. D_2 dopamine receptor binding in the basal ganglia of anti-psychotic free schizophrenic patients. A ^{123}I-IBZM single photon emission study. *Br J Psychiat* 1994; 164: 16–26.
(9) Stocklin G. Tracers for metabolic imaging of brain and heart: radiochemistry and radiopharmacology. *Eur J Nucl Med* 192; 19: 527–51.
(10) Savic I, Roland P, Sedvall G, Persson A, Paul S, Widen L. In vivo demonstration of reduced benzodiazepine receptor binding in human epileptic foci. *Lancet* 1988; ii: 863–6.
(11) Pilowsky LS, Costa DC, Ell PJ, Verhoeff NPLG, Murray RM, Kerwin RW. Antipsychotic medication, D_2 dopamine receptor blockade and clinical response: a ^{123}I-IBZM SPET (single photon emission tomography) study. *Psychol Med* 1993; 23: 791–7.
(12) Woods SW, Seibyl JP, Goddard AW et al. Dynamic SPECT imaging after injection of the benzodiazepine receptor ligand [^{123}I]iomazenil in healthy human subjects. *Psychiat Res: Neuroimaging* 1992; 45: 67–77.
(13) Seibyl JP, Woods SW, Zoghbi SS et al. Dynamic SPECT imaging of dopamine D2 receptors in human subjects with iodine-IBZM. *J Nucl Med* 1992; 33: 1964–71.
(14) Laruelle M, Abi-Dargham A, Rattner Z et al. Single photon emission tomography measurement of benzodiazepine receptor number and affinity in primate brain: a constant infusion paradigm with [^{123}I]iomazenil. *Eur J Pharmacol* 1993; 230: 119–23
(15) Pilowsky LS, Costa DC, Ell PJ, Murray RM, Verhoeff NPLG, Kerwin RW. Clozapine, single photon emission tomography and the D2 dopamine receptor blockade hypothesis of schizophrenia. *Lancet* 1992; ii: 199–202.
(16) Nyberg S, Farde L, Eriksson L, Halldin C, Eriksson B. $5HT_2$ and D_2 dopamine receptor occupancy in the living human brain. *Psychopharmacology* 1993; 110: 265–72.
(17) Seeman P, Lee T, Chau Wong M, Wong K. Antipsychotic drug doses and neuroleptic/dopamine receptors. *Nature* 1976; 261: 717–19.
(18) Crow TJ. Two syndromes in schizophrenia? *Trends Neurosci* 1982; 5: 351–4.
(19) Owen F, Crow TJ, Poulter M. Increased dopamine receptor sensitivity in schizophrenia. *Lancet* 1978; ii: 223–5.
(20) Wong DF, Wagner HN, Tune LE et al. Positron emission tomography reveals elevated D2 dopamine receptors in drug-naive schizophrenics. *Science* 1986; 234: 1558–63.
(21) Farde L, Wiesel F-A, Stone-Elander S et al. D2 dopamine receptors in neuroleptic-naive schizophrenic patients. A positron emission tomography study with [^{11}C]raclopride. *Arch Gen Psychiat* 1990; 47: 213–19.
(22) Martinot J-L, Pailliere-Martinot ML, Loc'h C et al. The estimated density of D2 striatal receptors in schizophrenia – a study with positron emission tomography and ^{76}Br bromolisuride. *Br J Psychiat* 1991; 158: 346–50.
(23) Gur RE, Resnick SM, Alavi A et al. Regional brain function in schizophrenia.

I. A positron emission tomography study. *Arch Gen Psychiat* 1987; 44: 119–25.
(24) Liddle PF, Friston KJ, Frith CD, Hirsch SR, Jones T, Frackowiak RSJ. Patterns of cerebral blood flow in schizophrenia. *Br J Psychiat* 1992; 160: 179–86.
(25) Meltzer HY, Stockmeier CA. In vivo occupancy of dopamine receptors by antipsychotic drugs. *Arch Gen Psychiat* 1992; 49: 588–9.
(26) Farde L, Nordström DL, Wiesel F, Pauli S, Halldin G, Sedvall G. Positron emission tomographic analysis of central D_1 and D_2 dopamine receptor occupancy in patients treated with classical neuroleptics and clozapine: relation to extrapyramidal side effects. *Arch Gen Psychiat* 1992; 49: 589–99.
(27) Kessler RM, Mason NS, Votaw JR et al. Visualization of extrastriatal dopamine D2 receptors in the human brain. *Eur J Pharmacol* 1993; 223: 105–7.
(28) Nordström A-L, Farde L, Wiesel F-A et al. Central D2-dopamine receptor occupancy in relation to antipsychotic drug effects: a double-blind PET study of schizophrenic patients. *Biol Psychiat* 1993; 33: 227–35.
(29) Busatto GF, Pilowsky LS, Costa DC, Ell PJ Verhoeff NPLG, Kerwin RW. Dopamine D2 receptor blockade in vivo with the novel atypical antipsychotics risperidone and remoxipride: a ^{123}I-IBZM SPET study. *Psychopharmacology* 1994 (in press).
(30) Kerwin RW. How do the neuropathological changes of schizophrenia relate to pre-existing neurotransmitter and aetiological hypothesis? *Psychol Med* 1989; 19: 563–7.
(31) Reynolds GP, Czudek C, Andrews HB. Deficit and hemispheric asymmetry of GABA reuptake sites in the hippocampus in schizophrenia. *Biol Psychiat* 1990; 27: 103–44.
(32) Benes FM, Vicent SL, Alsterberg G, Bird ED, SanGiovanni JP. Increased $GABA_A$ receptor binding in superficial layers of cingulate cortex in schizophrenics. *J Neurosci* 1992; 12: 924–9.
(33) Meldrum BS. Epilepsy and γ-aminobutyric acid-mediated inhibition. *Int Rev Neurobiol* 1975; 17: 1–36.
(34) Henry TR, Frey KA, Sackellares JC et al. In vivo cerebral metabolism and central benzodiazepine-receptor binding in temporal lobe epilepsy. *Neurology* 1993; 43: 1998–2006.
(35) Savic I, Ingvar M, Stone-Elander S. Comparison of [^{11}C]flumazenil and [^{18}F]FDG as PET markers of epileptic foci. *J Neurol, Neurosurg Psychiat* 1993; 56: 615–21.
(36) Cordes M, Henkes H, Ferstl F et al. Evaluation of focal epilepsy: a SPECT scanning comparison of ^{123}I-iomazenil versus HM-PAO. *Am J Neuroradiol* 1992; 13: 249–53.
(37) Bartenstein P, Ludolph A, Schober O et al. Benzodiazepine receptors and cerebral blood flow in partial epilepsy. *Eur J Nucl Med* 1991; 18: 111–18.
(38) Costa DC. Single photon emission tomography (SPET) with ^{99}Tc^{m}-hexamethylpropyleneamineoxime (HMPAO) in research and clinical practice – a useful tool. *Vasc Med Rev* 1990; 1: 179–201.
(39) Savic I, Thorell JO. PET shows different pattern of benzodiazepine receptor

changes in intractable compared with moderate partial epilepsy. *J Cereb Blood Flow Metab* 1993; 13 (suppl 1): S278.
(40) Savic I, Widen L, Thorell JO, Blomqvist G, Ericson K, Roland P. Cortical benzodiazepine receptor binding in patients with generalized and partial epilepsy. *Epilepsia* 1990; 31: 724–30.
(41) Rossor MN, Garrett NJ, Johnson AL, Mountjoy CQ, Roth M, Iversen LL. A post-mortem study of the cholinergic and GABA systems in senile dementia. *Brain* 1982; 105: 313–30.
(42) Blass JP. Pathophysiology of the Alzheimer's syndrome. *Neurology* 1993; 43 (suppl 4): S25–38.
(43) Weinberger DR, Gibson R, Coppola R et al. The distribution of cerebral muscarinic acetylcholine receptors in vivo in patients with dementia. A controlled study with ^{123}IQNB and single photon emission computed tomogrpahy. *Arch Neurol* 1991; 48: 169–76.
(44) Frackowiak RSJ, Pozzilli C, Legg NJ et al. Regional cerebral oxygen supply and utilization in dementia. A clinical and physiological study with oxygen-15 and positron emission tomography. *Brain* 1981; 104: 753–78.
(45) Burns A, Philpot MP, Costa DC, Ell PJ, Levy R. The investigation of Alzheimer's disease with single photon emission tomography. *J Neurol, Neurosurg Psychiat* 1989; 52: 248–53.
(46) Wyper DJ, Brown D, Patterson J, Owens J, Hunter R, McCulloch J. Density of acetylcholine receptors in Alzheimer's disease measured in relation to regional cerebral blood flow. *J Cereb Blood Flow Metab* 1993; 13 (suppl 1): S1.
(47) Blin J, Baron J-C, Dubois B et al. Loss of brain 5-HT2 receptors in Alzheimer's disease. *Brain* 1993; 116: 497–510.
(48) Volkow ND, Fowler JS, Wolf AP. Use of positron emission tomography to study cocaine in the human brain. In: Rapaka RS, Makriyannis A, Kuhar MJ, eds. *Emerging technologies and new directions in drug abuse research.* Rockville, MA: National Institute on Drug Abuse; 1991: 168–79.
(49) Volkow ND, Fowler JS, Wolf AP et al. Effects of chronic cocaine abuse on postsynaptic dopamine receptors. *Am J Psychiat* 1990; 147: 719–24.
(50) Volkow ND, Fowler JS, Wang GJ et al. Decreased dopamine D2 availability is associated with reduced frontal metabolism in cocaine abusers. *Synapse* 1993; 14: 169–77.
(51) Litton JE, Neiman J, Pauli S et al. PET analysis of [^{11}C]flumazenil binding to benzodiazepine receptors in chronic alcohol-dependent men and healthy controls. *Psychiat Res: Neuroimaging* 1993; 50: 1–13.
(52) Heninger GR, Charney DS. Mechanism of action of antidepressant treatments: implications for the etiology and treatment of depressive disorders. In: Meltzer HY, ed. *Psychopharmacolgy: the third generation of progress.* New York: Raven Press; 1987: 535–44.
(53) Meltzer HY, Lowy MT. The serotonin hypothesis of depression. In: Meltzer HY, ed. *Psychopharmacology: the third generation of progress.* New York: Raven Press; 1987: 513–26.
(54) Braestrup C, Nielsen M. Anxiety. *Lancet* 1982; ii; 1030–4.
(55) Hallstrom C. Benzodiazepines: clinical practice and central mechanisms. In:

Granville-Grossman, K, ed. *Recent advances in clinical psychiatry number 5*. London: Churchill Livingstone; 1985: 143–59.
(56) Feistel H, Kaschka WP, Ebert D, Joraschky P, Wolf F. Assessment of cerebral benzodiazepine receptor distribution in anxiety disorders – a study with ^{123}I-iomazenil. *J Nucl Med* 1993; 34 (suppl 5): 47 pp.
(57) Gray JA. Anxiety as a paradigm case of emotion. *Br Med Bull* 1981; 37: 193–7.
(58) Baxter LR, Schwartz JM, Mazziotta JC, Phelps ME, Pahl JJ, Guze BH. Cerebral glucose metabolic rates in nondepressed patients with obsessive–compulsive disorder. *Am J Psychiat* 1989; 145: 1560–3.
(59) Machlin SR, Harris GJ, Pearson GD, Hoehn-Saric R, Jeffery P, Camargo EE. Elevated medial-frontal cerebral blood flow in obsessive–compulsive patients: a SPECT study. *Am J Psychiat* 1991; 148: 1240–2.
(60) Murphy DL, Zohar J, Benkelfat C, Pato MT, Pigott TA, Insel TR. Obsessive–compulsive disorder as a 5-HT subsystem-related behavioural disorder. *Br J Psychiat* 1989; 155 (suppl 8): 15–24.
(61) Bonner TI. The molecular basis of muscarinic receptor diversity. *Trends Neurosci* 1989; 12: 148–51.
(62) Sibley DR, Monsma Jr FJ. Molecular biology of dopamine receptors. *Trends Pharmacol Sci* 1992; 13: 61–9.

Functional magnetic resonance imaging for psychiatry

R HOWARD and A DAVID

Magnetic resonance images are derived from nuclear magnetic resonance in which nuclear spins aligned by a uniform magnetic field are resonantly excited by a radiofrequency field. Strong magnetic fields are applied across the region to be imaged, and individual points within that region are identified by different resonance frequencies[1,2].

In all MRI techniques, the two-dimensional inverse Fourier transform of the MR image (known as the k-space) is sampled. Most MR images are formed using the spin–echo pulse sequence. Data sampling must be performed within a limited time period since the detected echo signal only lasts for 50–200 ms after each excitatory radiofrequency pulse. This process is known as T2 relaxation. Between excitations, a period of time (known as the repetition time or TR) must be allowed to pass in order for spins to return to alignment with the large static magnetic field imposed by the scanning machine. This process is called T1 relaxation. T1 relaxation is slow and time consuming and takes typically from 500 to 2000 ms.

There are two principal ways in which time taken for the acquisition of MR images can be reduced significantly.

If only very small radiofrequency pulses are used to excite a small fraction of the equilibrium magnetization, the time taken for TR may be cut to less than 100 ms and the echoes from which images will be created can be formed by a field gradient reversal as in the fast MRI techniques of FLASH and GRASS[1,2]. These images are generally T2* weighted, where T2* is the 'apparent T2' in the presence of magnetic field inhomogeneity.

Echo-planar imaging (EPI) involves a sampling strategy that is radically different from conventional MRI for which the acquisition of each line within the sampled space requires a fresh spin excitation. In EPI a single spin excitation is used to sample all of the image by generating up to 256

All correspondence to: Dr R Howard, Department of Psychiatry of Old Age, Institute of Psychiatry, De Crespigny Park, Denmark Hill, London SE5 9AF, UK.

Cambridge Medical Reviews: Neurobiology and Psychiatry Volume 3

echoes during the period of a single free induction decay. Data acquisition adequate to form a whole image can thus be completed in 50–100 ms. Because more use is made of the available spin magnetization than in conventional fast MRI, this improves the signal-to-noise ratio but the image is more vulnerable to distortions produced by magnetic field inhomogeneity[1,2].

The capacity of fast and ultra-fast MR imaging techniques for acquiring good quality images with high spatial resolution in less than a single second was welcomed initially for its potential both to cut down scanning times and reduce distortion of images by movement. Much more exciting than these qualities, however, is the capability for functional imaging that these techniques hold. Rather like the individual frames of a cine film, sequential images acquired in tens of milliseconds can follow the movements of solid structures such as the chambers of the heart in diastole and systole or the passage of extrinsic or intrinsic paramagnetic contrast agents within the vasculature.

Blood oxygenation-level dependent contrast imaging (BOLD)

Paramagnetic contrast agents such as Gadolinium have been used to image blood vessels with conventional MR for several years. Bolus injection of Gadolinium provided (as we shall see) the first functional MR maps of cortical activation[3]. Use of such extrinsic contrast agents has now been largely superseded by the totally non-invasive BOLD technique, originally developed in animals[4] and applied successfully to humans[5–7].

Since deoxyhaemoglobin contains paramagnetic iron, and oxygenated haemoglobin contains diamagnetic iron, changes in the relative concentrations of oxy- and deoxyhaemoglobin are readily detectable by MRI[4,8]. In effect, what happens is that signal strength increases as the relative concentration of deoxyhaemoglobin is reduced.

Neuronal activity within the brain results in local changes in cerebral blood flow, volume and oxygenation. In response to neuronal activation, local cerebral blood flow and volume increase so that oxygen delivery may increase by two to four times, yet oxygen extraction from blood increases only slightly[9]. Such an overcompensation of the vascular system to the local oxygen demands of active brain tissue means that the level of deoxyhaemoglobin in the capillaries and venules that drain an active focus actually is reduced. Increased neuronal activity during an activation task, therefore, will be reflected by a local increase in signal on T2* weighted images[10,11].

The properties of the BOLD signal enhancement, which is seen with neuronal activation, will be considered in more detail later. Briefly, there is a considerable latency of activation-induced BOLD signal change in primary cortical regions of 5–8 s from stimulus onset to the appearance of 90% of the maximum signal value and 5–9 s from stimulus cessation to return to

10% above signal baseline. Other, as yet unexplained, characteristics of BOLD are an 'undershoot' in signal after activation, decrease in baseline values after the first activation during cyclical or repeated activation and an occasional decrease in signal in some cortical regions observed during activation. Although the concept underlying BOLD may be simple, we still know very little about the delay, consistency, extent and incremental sensitivity of the in vivo vascular response to neuronal activation or the precise relationship between MRI signal enhancement and details of the pixel by pixel distribution of haemoglobin oxygenation, blood volume and vessel geometry.

Fast low angle shot (FLASH) and echo-planar imaging (EPI)

Since functional MRI studies follow the time course of oxy- and deoxyhaemoglobin-related signal changes within capillaries and venules, suitable approaches need to be both sensitive to focal inhomogeneities in the brain and rapid with respect to data acquisition. Rapid gradient echo imaging, in which gradient-recalled echoes formed by the application of a dephasing and rephasing magnetic field gradient are acquired, satisfies both these requirements and is used in both FLASH and EPI.

Typical FLASH sequences employ 64–256 radiofrequency (RF) pulses with flip angles smaller than 90 degrees, repetition times (TR) which are shorter than relaxation times (T1) and acquisition of at least one phase-encoded gradient echo per TR interval.

Single-shot EPI requires the application of only one 90-degree RF pulse followed by multiple reversals of the frequency-encoding read gradient. EPI is thus most advantageous when very short measuring times, of typically less than 100 ms, are required.

The other principal advantages of FLASH are the great flexibility of temporal and spatial resolution which it affords.

FLASH is commonly available as a two-dimensional and three-dimensional Fourier imaging technique on conventional MRI systems and is thus accessible in most centres. FLASH sequences may be used to unravel the mechanisms that underlie stimulus-related signal changes in functional MRI. For example, to what extent the intensities of points on activation maps refer to alterations of blood flow or deoxyhaemoglobin concentrations or both. FLASH sequences have the potential to discriminate between flow and deoxyhaemoglobin concentration effects by adjusting T1 and T2* contrasts via sequence parameters. Flow effects are emphasized by the combination of short echo times (for example, around 6 ms) and strong T1 saturation (for example, flip angles of 40 degrees and TRs of 40 ms). Sequences using RF pulses with very low flip angles to reduce flow-induced contributions to activation maps and long echo times permit deoxyhaemoglobin concentration change mapping.

Echo-planar imaging depends on a very rapidly switched magnetic field gradient of large amplitude and a fast capture of data. Since these expensive features are not necessary in commercially produced MR systems, only certain specialist centres have echo-planar capability.

Echo-planar imaging is extremely fast. For brain imaging, with equivalent voxel size, an EPI image with an acquisition time of 40 ms will have the same signal-to-noise ratio as a FLASH image which takes 2 s to acquire. Faster FLASH images will thus have a poorer signal-to-noise ratio than echo-planar images. Since a complete echo-planar image is acquired in under 100 ms, motion artefact from whole patient movement, or arterial and CSF pulsations, is eliminated.

The echo-planar technique normally uses a full 90-degree RF pulse or spin excitation, thus providing a high single shot signal-to-noise ratio. A further advantage of 90-degree flip angle EPI, using a TR of 1–3 s, is that many slices of the subject can be acquired rapidly in an interleaved manner. Up to 15 slices per second can be imaged, allowing a complete volume scan of the brain in around 2 s.

The major problems associated with the use of gradient–echo EPI with a long echo time arise from the very high sensitivity of the technique to inhomogeneities of the magnetic field. Anything less than ideal shimming results in severe signal loss. No amount of shimming can remove natural field gradients such as those produced at the air/brain interface around the sinuses. Brain areas close to sinuses and the petrous temporal bone hence suffer a degree of signal loss distortion. In addition, deep-lying structures such as the hippocampus and medial temporal lobe are poorly visualized by such sequences.

A second major problem affecting both FLASH and EPI gradient–echo sequences is that draining veins carrying hyperoxygenated blood away from areas of activation will have a major effect on the MR signal near them which may bear no functional relation to the performed task. Spin–echo (SE) sequences can go some way towards overcoming this problem. Spin–echo EPI, for example, has the potential to discriminate active cortical areas from draining veins. At high field strengths of around 4 T, veins have very low intensity on SE images with a TE of greater than 40 ms. Vessels of less than 30 microns in diameter dominate contrast changes on such sequences while gradient–echo (GE) images are sensitive to changes in vessels of any diameter. Thus, the differences between SE and GE images can be used to pinpoint draining veins.

Functional MRI and cortical activation mapping

Developments in fMRI that are potentially the most exciting for psychiatrists are the elegant and non-invasive measures of cortical activation evoked by neuropsychological paradigms that involve sensory stimulation, the generation of motor or verbal outputs and more abstract mental processes such as imagery. What follows is by no means a complete catalogue of extant studies of this kind, but intends to give a flavour of what fMRI has been able to do in the investigation of cortical activation.

Visual cortex

The first demonstration of cortical activation in response to visual stimulation has been mentioned already[3]. Two boluses of Gadolinium were given to subjects; one at rest in a darkened room and the second during full-field visual stimulation. Sixty images were obtained over a 45-s period with each EPI image acquired in 64 ms. Increases in rCBF of at least 20% were seen in all of seven subjects, and these blood flow changes were overlayed on to three-dimensional surface-rendered MR scans with impressive anatomic localization of the striate cortex.

Application of BOLD to activation mapping of visual cortex has been very successful. Using flashing checker-board photic stimulation on the screen of an LCD projection television, Kwong et al[12] measured mean changes on activation of 2.5% in the T2* weighted gradient–echo signal in areas V1 and V2. Using EPI with a scanning time of 100 ms, a spatial resolution of $1.5 \times 1.5 \times 3.0$ mm was attained. Extrastriate cortical activation in area V5 was also detected in some subjects. Turner et al[13] measured variations in image intensity in V1 of 28% at 4 T and 7% at 1.5 T with photic stimulation using gradient–echo EPI.

Crude retinotopic mapping of V1 was initially investigated by measurement of activation during alternating hemifield activation with a black and white counterphase 8 Hz semiannular checker-board[14]. Activation was measured with both a gradient–echo sequence sensitive to changes in T2* and a T1-sensitive (blood flow) spin–echo inversion–recovery sequence with a resolution of $1.5 \times 1.5 \times 3.0$ mm. Left and right visual fields were alternately stimulated every 50 s and the dynamic changes seen in cortical activation in left and right V1 areas exactly followed the reversal frequency.

The retinotopic organization of the visual cortex has been investigated in much greater detail with these techniques. In one study[15], while subjects fixated on a white dot on a uniform black video projector screen, black and white checkered rings centred on the fixation point of varying sizes were presented for 10 s. EPI images were acquired and foci of brain activation were demonstrated within V1 and in additional sites on the medial brain surface (including V2) and the posterior wall of the parieto-occipital sulcus. Within the calcarine fissure, increasing the degree of eccentricity of the checkered ring from the fixation point led to an anterior progression of activity from the occipital pole. These authors acknowledged that reconstruction of the infolded cortical mantle buried within the calcarine sulcus would be necessary before detailed maps can be produced and such 'cortical ribbon mapping' has in fact been reported only extremely recently. Ingenious development of computer algorithms, which control for individual subjects' unique folding of the cortex to produce a flattened cortical ribbon along which activation patterns can be mapped, has been an important advance[16]. Using a conventional 1.5 T scanner and a T2* gradient–echo sequence, Scheider et al[16] have been able to distinguish four topographically distinct areas along such a cortical ribbon from the striate cortex. Activation of each of the four areas corresponded with the four types of visual field stimulation used (left–right, top–bottom).

Brain activation maps calculated with actual photic stimulation have been compared with those obtained when a subject is asked to recall mental images of the same stimulus[17]. Light-proof goggles fitted with red light-emitting diodes geometrically arranged as two square patterns which flash at 16 Hz were used for a 30-s prestimulation of the visual cortex during which subjects were asked to memorize the stimulus. The stimulus was then switched alternately off and on for further periods of 30 s and, during the off periods, subjects were asked to imagine the previously seen stimulus. Coronal EPI images were acquired, perpendicular to the calcarine fissure. Areas of maximum response to stimulation occurred in 10–20 mm^2 regions of interest in areas V1 and V2. During photic stimulation, the bilateral increase in MR signal averaged 2.8% in seven subjects. In five of these individuals, signal increases averaging 1.5% in the same regions were seen while recalling the image. Hence, changes associated with cognition such as the mental representation of an imagined visual pattern can be mapped non-invasively in real time with good spatial resolution using fMRI. The authors concluded from their results that, during early recollection, mental images may be formed not only from stored representations but by an active reconstruction process utilizing topographically mapped cortical areas involved in early visual processing.

With more imaginative and complex material for visual mental imagery, Menon et al[18] used a FLASH system with 5-s image acquisition and 40 ms echo time to detect activation while subjects imagined performing a navigational task amongst familiar scenery, or imagined individual familiar objects such as fruits and vegetables. The imagined navigational task induced signal changes of 3% to 7% in the parieto-occipital sulcus in addition to changes in V1, while imagining familiar objects induced small changes in those V1 regions where large signal changes had been observed during photic stimulation.

Functional coupling of cortical and subcortical components of the visual system has been demonstrated with these techniques. By acquiring a T1 weighted FLASH sequence orientated parallel to the bicommissural plane, Frahm et al[19] included both the lateral geniculate nucleus and primary visual cortex in the same image. The temporal pattern of hyperoxygenated phases detected in response to binocular stimulation at 10 Hz were identical in both the primary visual cortex and the lateral geniculate nucleus.

Motor cortex

When subjects are asked to tap each finger against the ipsilateral thumb, the signal change detected from primary motor cortex remains stable, even for prolonged activations of up to 6 min[20]. When the duration of activation is altered from 0.5 s to 5 s, the pattern of signal enhancement observed is remarkably constant, beginning 2–3 s after activation onset and continuing for 3–5 s before reaching baseline again[20].

Functional localization within the primary and supplementary motor cortex has been the subject of more detailed study. Using a gradient–echo EPI sequence with a 40 ms acquisition time and a TR of 2 s, Rao et al[15] examined activation of both the primary (Brodmann area 4) and secondary (supplementary motor area and premotor cortex of Brodmann area 6) motor cortex. Subjects were asked to perform a simple motor task in which they tapped their fingers as fast as they could, and a complex task in which they tapped four fingers in a fixed and repeating sequence. The simple task activated the contralateral primary motor cortex alone, while the complex task produced activation in primary motor cortex, supplementary motor area, premotor and somatosensory areas. When subjects were asked to imagine the finger movements, activation was seen in the supplementary motor area. The authors concluded that their results supported a hierarchical model of voluntary motor control and that fMRI is able to demonstrate higher order mental processing in the absence of primary sensory stimulation or motor activation. Other authors[21] have confirmed that the observed regions of increased signal intensity seen for imagining and performing tasks are essentially the same, although performance induces a greater degree of change than mental rehearsal.

Somatotopic mapping of the primary motor cortex with echo-planar imaging has been able to distinguish clearly between cortical activation accompanying finger, elbow, tongue and toe movements, and the cortical areas activated by such voluntary movements were generally similar in spatial topography to those derived from stimulation studies[22].

Auditory cortex and language

Initial studies using gradient–echo EPI showed 1.5–2.4% increases in signal intensity from the superior temporal gyrus during passive word presentation[23]. Superior spatial resolution and the ability to generate images based on repeated measurements of single individuals mean that fMRI can extend our knowledge of functional anatomy by increasing the level of detail in which anatomic areas can be examined. The superior temporal sulcus and anatomically closely located regions such as the planum temporale, which are difficult to separate with PET or lesioning experiments, may play particular parts in processing auditory sensory input. To investigate this with EPI, symmetrical lateral sagittal slices were acquired of the left and right hemispheres centred at positions 8 mm medial to the most lateral point of the temporal lobe on each side[15]. Auditory stimuli (louder than machine noise) were delivered via air-filled tubes to headphones. White noise stimulation produced signal increases which were confined to the dorsal aspect of the superior temporal gyrus and the lateral aspect of the transverse temporal gyrus. Activation responses to speech involved a wider area which included the dorsal superior temporal gyrus and the superior temporal sulcus. The activation area tended to be largest when subjects were presented with nonsense 'pseudowords' such as narb, orsh or skob. Turner et al[13] provided auditory stimulation with a single musical note (G or 1680 Hz) at sufficient volume for it to be heard by subjects over the noise of an echo-planar machine (1000 Hz). Areas of activation were observed in the regions reported by Rao et al[23] for white noise and speech.

In an investigation of cortical activation accompanying word generation and internal speech[24,25], subjects performed silent, self-paced word generation from each of the letters of the alphabet without physical articulation or vocalization. Axial images of the perisylvian region including the left inferior frontal gyrus (Broca's area) and its right-sided homologue were acquired using a T2* weighted gradient–echo FLASH sequence. Lateralized activation of Broca's area was clearly demonstrated during task performance with a brisk rise in signal intensity and subsequent return to baseline. This lateralization is in accord with earlier PET studies which have suggested that word generation tasks are accompanied by exclusively left-sided frontal activation[26,27].

With a result that begs to be repeated and which differs importantly from the PET work, McCarthy et al[28] have demonstrated that the frontal activation which occurs during a word generation task may be bilateral. Using EPI to acquire a 1 cm thick axial slice 0.8 cm below the anterior commissure–posterior commissure (AC–PC) line projected into the frontal lobes, subjects were scanned at rest, making lip movements, listening to presented words, repeating presented words and generating verbs to match presented nouns. Little or no activation was observed during resting, listening or motor periods, but during verb generation a mean fractional signal change of 10.5% occurred. Activation occurred within 3 s of task onset and could be observed in single images from individual subjects. The primary focus of activation was left frontal grey matter along a sulcus anterior to the lateral sulcus, including the anterior insula, Brodmann area 47 and extending to area 10. Significant activation was also seen in a homologous region in the right frontal cortex.

'Covert performance' of a word generation task, in which the subject generates words internally but does not pronounce them, appears to utilize the same cortical areas as overt performance. Rueckert et al[29] examined subjects who had been asked to generate as many words as possible beginning with a particular letter with gradient–echo EPI. All subjects showed activation in Broca's area, and significant activation was also detected in motor and premotor cortex in a region corresponding to the face area.

Memory

Primate lesion and human PET studies have suggested that the dorsolateral prefrontal cortex, in particular Brodmann areas 9 and 46, is the neuronal source of memory for the location of objects in the visual field. In a fMRI investigation of 'working memory', or the capacity to keep a running record of ongoing events, EPI images of a 1 cm coronal slice passing through areas 9 and 46 were acquired during performance of a spatial working memory task[30]. A series of novel shapes were presented in any of 12 locations on an LCD panel computer projection system. A 'sensory memory' task consisted of instructing subjects to make a finger movement if they saw a stimulus that was red in colour, while 'location memory' was tested by asking subjects to make finger movements if any stimulus appeared in a previously occupied location on the screen. Activation generated by both tasks was centred on area 9, and the greatest degree of activation was seen with the location memory task.

The dorsolateral prefrontal cortex and inferior surface of the middle frontal gyrus were the most reliable areas of activation during a further working memory task[31]. Subjects were asked to watch for a repeating sequence of letters on a video display and to respond only when the current letter was the same as the letter two back. During the control situation, subjects again watched letters on a screen and responded when a particular letter, such as the letter X, appeared.

Neuropsychiatric conditions

At the time of writing, functional MRI has been confined largely to investigations of physiological, rather than pathological, brain function. There are a few isolated exceptions to this, however. An increase in signal intensity (following the injection of a bolus of Gadolinium) has been recorded from V1 during photic stimulation of patients with mild to moderately severe Alzheimer's disease[32]. These authors concluded that degenerative brain disease does not appear to limit the potential usefulness of the technique.

Patients with either quadrantanopia or homonymous hemianopia stimulated with light-proof goggles flashing at 8 Hz showed a clear asymmetry in the degree of functional activation observed between the affected side and the clinically normal side[33]. Extrastriate activation, however, was similar on both sides, despite this marked asymmetry in striatal activation, and the authors suggest that this may indicate the neural activity responsible for the phenomenon of blindsight in which patients are able to appreciate motion without conscious visual perception.

In what must certainly be the first published fMRI studies of a *functional* psychiatric disorder, Breiter et al[34] observed signal intensity changes of 1.5–4% in the orbital gyri and dorsolateral prefrontal cortex of patients with obsessional–compulsive disorder during symptom provocation. This finding is similar to that reported in earlier PET studies and was not seen during disgust reactions induced in normal control subjects. What had not been shown with PET was the real time changes of cortical activation which began within 3 s of provocation and lasted throughout the scanning session. A further novel finding was variable signal changes recorded from the temporal lobes.

The pattern and intensity of activation observed during performance of a simple motor task, and during visual stimulation in schizophrenic patients and healthy controls in two reports to date, have demonstrated an apparently inconsistent effect of the illness and prescribed medication. (We can no doubt expect to see a flurry of such reports of apparent differences between schizophrenics and controls during a number of activation paradigms, but perhaps the most illuminating fMRI studies in this field will be those which focus more on activation accompanying psychopathological events.) In the first of these, when 10 right-handed schizophrenics and 10 healthy volunteers performed rapid sequential finger to thumb opposition, all subjects showed a significant activation in the contralateral and ipsilateral sensorimotor cortex[35]. Schizophrenic patients, however, showed a significantly reduced global activation strength compared with the volunteers. Selective evaluation of left-hand, compared with right-hand, movements indicated an increase in global activation in volunteers but a decrease in patients and a reduced co-activation in the dominant hemisphere was found in patients compared with controls during movement of the left hand. The authors concluded that these changes may be indicative of disturbed interhemispheric interaction in schizophrenia and that reduced levels of activation could be attributed to the combined effects of the disease and prescribed medication.

Quite the opposite effect has been reported in measures of activation in response to photic stimulation in schizophrenia[36]. Mean signal change in V1 was significantly greater in eight patients with schizophrenia (4.6%) than in nine healthy volunteers (3.1%).

Why is fMRI so applicable to psychiatric research?

The absolute non-invasiveness of fMRI compared with PET and SPET is the most obvious advantage that it holds. Potential for dispensing with injections of intravenous contrast and radioactive tracer or ligand will be greeted with relief by those researchers who spend their time persuading psychiatric patients to undergo functional imaging. Removal of any concern regarding radioactivity means that there is no theoretical limit to the number of repeated scans a subject may undergo. Thus, changes in brain activity accompanying learning, memory, mood or biochemical and hormonal fluctuations can be investigated over periods of days, weeks, months or even years. For psychological events that are rapid and sometimes short lived such as hallucinations, delusions, thought disorder and depersonalization experiences, underlying cortical activation can be mapped and followed during long sequences of frequently repeated image acquisitions.

The next apparent advantages over earlier functional brain imaging techniques are the superior spatial and temporal resolution of fMRI. Conventional PET and SPET images reveal brain activity over a time period of at least a minute and have spatial resolution of no better than 6 mm. The temporal resolution of fMRI in measuring the changes that accompany cortical activation would seem to be limited only by the physiological reactivity of regional cerebral blood flow to focal neuronal activity. The observed time delay of 3–8 s between onset of stimulation and haemodynamic response and the transient period of deoxygenation that follows activation act as a rate-limiting step, rather than any parameters associated with the technology, since acquisition of 14 images per second is possible[5].

A spatial resolution of functional activation maps that is 2 orders of magnitude better than that achievable by PET has been reported using gradient–echo FLASH sequences with a voxel size of 2.5 to 39 microlitres[37]. Two-dimensional in-plane resolution of as good as 1.3 × 2.0 mm is feasible[7]. Ultimately, spatial resolution is only limited by the extent to which magnetic field inhomogeneities outside capillaries and the smallest venules exceed the calibre of those vessels.

Not only can fMRI produce images with excellent spatial resolution, but these can be mapped on to brain contours derived from high resolution structural images acquired in the same plane and during the same scanning session. This offers a clear advantage over attempts to co-register images made during different imaging modalities such as PET and MRI.

A final advantageous feature of fMRI is that the degree of activation observed within a single subject is of such a significant magnitude that there is no need to average data acquired from several subjects. Few PET workers[38] have been able to produce a signal-to-noise ratio high enough to detect changes in single subjects.

Prospects

It is fortuitous that the cortical areas underpinning higher mental functions which have emerged time and again in this review are the dorsolateral prefrontal cortex, auditory association areas and Broca's area since these are the areas which have drawn most attention from psychiatric researchers investigating psychotic phenomena. Prefrontal cortex has been implicated in disorders of motivation and internal monitoring[39,40] which may underlie some of the negative symptoms of schizophrenia, such as lack of volition, and positive symptoms, such as thought alienation. The superior temporal gyrus, particularly on the left side, has been found to be abnormal on high resolution structural scanning of chronic schizophrenics, and correlations with key symptoms such as auditory hallucinations[41] and thought disorder[42] with reduced volumes of this region have been reported. Increased metabolism in Broca's area during auditory hallucinosis has also been demonstrated with PET techniques[43]. Functional MRI is thus poised to contribute further to our knowledge of these areas by virtue of its ability to capture such phenomena which may be transient and hence elusive.

While the urge to apply fMRI to psychiatric research may seem to be irresistible, we should not forget that valid and enduring studies will depend on a solid foundation of normative psychophysiological data. While auditory and visual hallucinations may seem an obvious topic for study with fMRI, this cannot be done definitively until we have a clear picture of the functional anatomy of perception and imagery such as is being sketched out with PET[44,45]. Close collaboration will be needed with cognitive and neuropsychologists, as well as with physicists and radiologists, if fMRI in psychiatry is to fulfil its undoubted potential.

Acknowledgement

We are particularly grateful to Martin Graves, Principal Physicist at St George's Hospital MR unit, for his comments on a draft of this chapter.

References

(1) Cohen MS, Weisskoff RM. Ultra-fast imaging. *Magn Res Imaging* 1991; 9: 1–37.
(2) Stehling MK, Turner R, Mansfield P. Echo-planar imaging: magnetic resonance imaging in a fraction of a second. *Science* 1991; 254: 43–50.
(3) Belliveau JW, Kennedy DN, McKinstry RC et al. Functional mapping of the human visual cortex by magnetic resonance imaging. *Science* 1991; 254: 716–19.
(4) Ogawa S, Lee T-M, Kay AR, Tank DW. Brain magnetic resonance imaging with contrast dependent blood oxygenation. *Proc Natl Acad Sci USA* 1990; 87: 9868–72.
(5) Bandettini PA, Wong EC, Hinks RS, Tikofsky RS, Hyde JSA. Time course EPI of human brain function during task activation. *Magn Res Med* 1992; 25: 390–7.

(6) Kwong KK, Belliveau JW, Chesler DA et al. Dynamic magnetic resonance imaging of human brain activity during primary sensory stimulation. *Proc Natl Acad Sci USA* 1992; 89: 5675–9.
(7) Ogawa S, Tank DW, Menon R, Ellerman JM, Kim SG, Merkle H, Urgurbil K. Intrinsic signal changes accompanying sensory stimulation: functional brain mapping with magnetic resonance imaging. *Proc Natl Acad Sci USA* 1992; 89: 5951–5.
(8) Turner R, Le Bihan D, Moonen CT, Despres D, Frank J. Echo-planar time course MRI of cat brain oxygenation changes. *Magn Res Med* 1991; 22: 159–66.
(9) Fox PT, Raichle ME. Focal physiological uncoupling of cerebral blood flow and oxidative metabolism during somatosensory stimulation in human subjects. *Proc Nat Acad Sci USA* 1986; 83: 1140–4.
(10) Ogawa S, Lee T-M. Magnetic resonance imaging of blood vessels at high fields: in vivo and in vitro measurements and image simulation. *Magn Res Med* 1990; 16: 9–18.
(11) Ogawa S, Lee T-M, Nayak AS, Glynn P. Oxygen-sensitive contrast in magnetic resonance image of rodent brain at high magnetic fields. *Magn Res Med* 1990; 14: 68–78.
(12) Kwong KK, Chesler DA, Baker JR et al. Functional magnetic resonance imaging – MR movie of human brain activity. Proceedings of the Society of Magnetic Resonance in Medicine, June 17–19, Arlington, Virginia, 1993: 135–42.
(13) Turner R, Jezzard P, Wen H et al. Functional mapping of the human visual cortex at 4 and 1.5 tesla using deoxygenation contrast EPI. *Magn Res Med* 1993; 29: 277–9.
(14) Belliveau JW, Kwong KK, Baker JR et al. MRI mapping of human visual cortex: retinotopic organisation and frequency of response of V1. Proceedings of the Society of Magnetic Resonance in Medicine, 8–14 August, Berlin, 1992: 310.
(15) Rao SM, Binder JR, DeYoe EA et al. Functional MRI studies of the human motor, auditory and visual cortices. Proceedings of the Society of Magnetic Resonance in Medicine, June 17–19, Arlington, Virginia, 1993; 197–205.
(16) Schneider W, Noll DC, Cohen JD. Functional topographic mapping of the cortical ribbon in human vision with conventional MRI scanners. *Nature* 1993; 365: 150–3.
(17) Le Bihan D, Turner R, Zeffiro TA et al. Activation of human primary visual cortex during mental imagery. Proceedings of the Society of Magnetic Resonance in Medicine, June 17–19, Arlington, Virginia, 1993: 191–6.
(18) Menon R, Ogawa S, Tank DW, Ellerman JM, Merkle H, Urgurbil K. Visual mental imagery by functional MRI. Proceedings of the Society of Magnetic Resonance in Medicine, 12th Meeting, 14–20 August, New York, 1993: 1381.
(19) Frahm J, Merboldt KD, Hanicke W, Kleinschmidt A, Steinmetz H. High-resolution functional MRI of focal subcortical activity in the human brain. Long-echo time FLASH of the lateral geniculate nucleus during visual stimulation. Proceedings of the Society of Magnetic Resonance in Medicine, 12th Annual Meeting, 14–20 August, New York, 1993: 57.
(20) Bandettini PA. MRI studies of brain activation: dynamic characteristics.

Proceedings of the Society of Magnetic Resonance in Medicine, June 17–19, Arlington, Virginia, 1993: 143–51.

(21) Feldman JB, Cohen LG, Jezzard P et al. Functional neuroimaging with echo-planar imaging in humans during execution and mental rehearsal of a simple motor task. Proceedings of the Society of Magnetic Resonance in Medicine, 12th Annual Meeting, 14–20 August, New York, 1993: 1416.

(22) Rao SM, Binder JR, Lisk LM et al. Somatotopic mapping of the primary motor cortex with functional magnetic resonance imaging. Proceedings of the Society of Magnetic Resonance in Medicine, 14–20 August, New York, 1993: 1397.

(23) Rao SM, Bandettini PA, Wong EC et al. Gradient–echo EPI demonstrates bilateral superior temporal gyrus activation during passive word presentation. Proceedings of the Society of Magnetic Resonance Imaging in Medicine, 8–14 August, Berlin, 1992: 1827.

(24) Hinke RM, Hu X, Stillman AE et al. Functional magnetic resonance imaging of Broca's area during internal speech. *NeuroReport* 1993; 4: 675–8.

(25) Hinke RM, Hu X, Stillman AE, Kim S-G, Urgurbil K. Multislice gradient-echo functional MRI of internal speech at 4 tesla. Proceedings of the Society of Magnetic Resonance in Medicine, 17–19 June, Arlington, Virginia, 1993: 251.

(26) Frith CD, Friston KJ, Liddle PF, Frackowiak RSJ. A PET study of word finding. *Neuropsychologica* 1991; 29: 1137–48.

(27) Petersen SE, Fox PT, Snyder AZ, Raichle ME. Activation of extrastriate and frontal cortical areas by visual words and word-like stimuli. *Science* 1990; 249: 1041–4.

(28) McCarthy G, Blamire AM, Rothman DL, Gruetter R, Shulman RG. Echo-planar magnetic resonance imaging studies of frontal cortex activation during word generation in humans. *Proc Natl Acad Sci USA* 1993; 90: 4952–6.

(29) Rueckert L, Appollonio I, Grafman J et al. Functional activation of left frontal cortex during covert word production. Proceedings of the Society of Magnetic Resonance in Medicine, 12th Annual Meeting, 14–20 August, New York, 1993: 60.

(30) Blamire AM, McCarthy G, Nobre AC et al. Functional magnetic resonance imaging during a spatial working memory task in humans. Proceedings of the Society of Magnetic Resonance in Medicine, 17–19 June, Arlington, Virginia, 1993: 250.

(31) Cohen JD, Forman SD, Casey BJ, Noll DC. Spiral-scan imaging of dorsolateral prefrontal cortex during a working memory task. Proceedings of the Society of Magnetic Resonance in Medicine, 12th Annual Meeting, 14–20 August, New York, 1993: 1405.

(32) Mattay VS, Frank JA, Sunderland T et al. Dynamic contrast functional MRI in Alzheimer's disease during visual activation. Proceedings of the Society of Magnetic Resonance in Medicine, 12th Annual Meeting, 14–20 August, New York, 1993: 1404.

(33) Sorensen AG, Carama F, Wray SH et al. Extrastriate activation in patients with visual field defects. Proceedings of the Society of Magnetic Resonance in Medicine, 12th Annual Meeting, 14–20 August, New York, 1993: 62.

(34) Breiter HC, Kwong KK, Baker JR et al. Functional magnetic resonance imaging of symptom provocation in obsessive–compulsive disorder. Proceedings of the Society of Magnetic Resonance in Medicine, 12th Annual Meeting, 14–20 August, New York, 1993: 58.

(35) Wenz F, Schad LR, Knopp MV et al. Functional magnetic resonance imaging at 1.5 T: activation pattern in schizophrenic patients receiving neuroleptic medication. *Magn Res Imaging* 1994; 12: 975–82.

(36) Renshaw PF, Yurgelun-Todd DA, Cohen B. Greater haemodynamic response to photic stimulation in schizophrenic patients: an echoplanar MRI study. *Am J Psychiat* 1994; 151: 1493–5.

(37) Frahm J, Merboldt K-D, Hanicke W. Functional MRI of human brain activation at high spatial resolution. *Magn Res Med* 1993; 29: 139–44.

(38) Watson JDG, Myers R, Frackowiak RSJ et al. Area V5 of the human brain: evidence from a combined study using positron emission tomography and magnetic resonance imaging. *Cereb Cortex* 1993; 3: 79–94.

(39) Frith CD, Done DJ. Towards a neuropsychology of schizophrenia. *Br J Psychiat* 1985; 153: 437–43.

(40) Weinberger DR, Breman KF, Suddath R, Torrey EF. Evidence of dysfunction of a prefrontal–limbic network in schizophrenia: a magnetic resonance imaging and regional cerebral blood flow study of discordant monozygotic twins. *Am J Psychiat* 1992; 149: 890–7.

(41) Barta PE, Pearlson GD, Powers RE, Richards SS, Tune LE. Auditory hallucinations and smaller superior temporal gyral volume in schizophrenia. *Am J Psychiat* 1990; 147: 1457–62.

(42) Shenton ME, Kikins R, Jolesz R et al. Abnormalities of the left temporal lobe and thought disorder in schizophrenia. *New Engl J Psychiat* 1992; 327: 604–12.

(43) Cleghorn JM, Franco S, Szechtman B et al. Towards a brain map of auditory hallucinations. *Am J Psychiat* 1992; 149: 1062–9.

(44) Kosslyn SM, Alpert NM, Thompson WL et al. Visual mental mental imagery activated topographically organised visual cortex: PET investigations. *J Cogn Neurosci* 1993; 5: 263–987.

(45) Paulesu E, Frith CD, Frackowiak RSJ. The neural correlates of the verbal component of working memory. *Nature* 1992; 362: 342–4.

PET studies of cerebral function in schizophrenia

P F LIDDLE

Positron emission tomography (PET) provides images of brain function that reveal that the pathophysiology of schizophrenia entails widespread disturbance of cerebral function, especially in the multimodal association cortical areas which serve the highest of human mental activities. However, interpretation of functional images is fraught with difficulty because of the many sources of variance between and within subjects. Some of these sources of variance, such as variation in cerebral activity with variation in concurrent mental activity, and variations in the pattern of neural activity associated with a specific mental process, are potentially informative provided appropriate comparisons are performed. Other sources of variance, such as variation in global flow or metabolism due to systemic metabolic fluctuations, and variations in brain orientation, size and shape, are potentially confounding and must be minimized. Hence, before reviewing the results of studies of schizophrenic patients, it is important to consider issues of imaging technique; study design; and strategies for allowing for potentially confounding variance.

PET techniques for imaging brain function

The images of brain function are obtained by tomographic reconstruction of the pattern of distribution in the brain of tracer substances whose distribution reflects either regional cerebral blood flow (rCBF) or glucose metabolism (rCMRglu). The tracer most commonly used for measuring rCBF is water labelled with the positron emitting isotope of oxygen (^{15}O). The usual tracer for rCMRglu is deoxyglucose labelled with the positron emitting isotope of fluorine (^{18}F). Images obtained using tracer substances labelled with ^{18}F have a slightly better spatial resolution because the positron emitted by ^{18}F has a lower energy than that emitted by ^{15}O and hence tends to travel

All correspondence to: Dr P F Liddle, Department of Psychiatry, University of British Columbia, 2255 Wesbrook Mall, Vancouver, Canada V6T 2A1.

Cambridge Medical Reviews: Neurobiology and Psychiatry Volume 3

a shorter distance before it is annihilated to generate the pair of photons that are detected by the PET camera.

However, images of rCBF obtained using $H_2{}^{15}O$ are potentially much more informative about brain function than images of rCMRglu for two reasons. First, rCBF is a more sensitive indicator of changes in neural activity than rCMRglu. Studies using magnetic resonance imaging (MRI) with a fast pulse sequence capable of imaging the change in paramagnetism of blood due to the change in the ratio of oxyhaemoglobin to deoxyhaemoglobin associated with neural activity, indicate that there is a reflex local increase in rCBF over a time scale of several seconds after neurones become active, and that this increase in rCBF is greater than that required to meet the increased metabolic demand[1].

Secondly, because ^{15}O has a half-life of only 2.1 minutes, scans can be repeated after about 10 minutes, and it is possible to obtain images of up to 12 different brain states in an individual subject during a single scanning session. As equilibrium between the concentration of $H_2{}^{15}O$ in tissue and the concentration in the blood perfusing that tissue is achieved within seconds, a rCBF image reflects the pattern of cerebral activity at the time of arrival of the labelled water in the brain. If the $H_2{}^{15}O$ is administered as a bolus infusion over a period of 30 seconds, the image reflects brain activity averaged over a period of similar duration. The ability to obtain multiple images in a single subject makes it possible to explore changes in cerebral activity associated with performance of cognitive tasks; to establish the relationship between variations in neural activity in different cerebral areas; and also to study the influence of pharmacological agents on cerebral function.

In contrast, ^{18}F has a half-life of 118 minutes so scans cannot be repeated in a single scanning session. The accumulation of deoxyglucose in brain cells occurs over a time scale of approximately 30 minutes, so it is necessary to sustain the brain state of interest for that period of time. Therefore, the ^{18}F-deoxyglucose technique for imaging rCMRglu is useful mainly for studying patterns of cerebral activity associated with stable mental states, or relatively slowly changing pharmacological effects.

Although this review will focus principally upon PET studies of cerebral function, it is also possible to image rCBF using single photon emission tomography (SPET) with the tracer HMPAO labelled with the metastable photon emitting isotope ^{99m}Tc. The concentration of ^{99m}Tc-HMPAO in tissue reaches a rapid equilibrium with that in blood, so that the image reflects cerebral activity within a few seconds after the labelled tracer in the brain. However, the very long half-life of ^{99m}Tc not only results in greater radiation exposure but also makes it impossible to obtain independent scans in a single scanning session. Some investigators use a split-dose technique in which half of the dose is administered during a second brain state, after the first image has been recorded. An image of the second brain state can be derived by subtracting the estimated radioactivity due to the first half of dose of ^{99m}Tc-HMPAO from the final distribution of radioactivity.

Design of functional imaging studies

rCBF and rCMRglu depend on current neuronal activity which, in turn, depends upon concurrent mental activity. Not surprisingly, studies which have used PET to compare schizophrenic subjects with control subjects without considering the specific mental state during scanning have yielded rather confusing results. It is necessary to design functional imaging studies in a way that allows comparison between images recorded in mental states that differ with regard to the aspect of mental processing which is of interest.

There are two types of approach to the design of studies. The first approach is the categorical approach and entails comparison of images obtained during a mental state of interest with images obtained in an appropriate reference state. The second approach is the correlational approach and entails a series of scans in a variety of different mental states that involve the aspect of mental processing of interest to varying degrees. The object of analysis is to identify the pixels in which there is a significant correlation between cerebral activity and the degree of involvement in the mental process of interest. In both, the categorical approach and the correlational approach, it is desirable to perform within-subject comparisons, though in situations where the different mental states of interest cannot be achieved within an individual subject, it is necessary to perform comparisons between different mental states in different subjects.

Cerebral activity associated with symptom expression

If the object is to determine the pattern of cerebral activity associated with the expression of a particular symptom, either the categorical or correlational design might be employed. In the categorical approach, rCBF in the presence of the symptom would be compared with rCBF in the absence of the symptom. If there is variation in other aspects of the mental state, apart from the symptom of interest, between the pairs of images, it is necessary to perform a covariance analysis to allow for variation in the potentially confounding variables. In the correlational approach (across subjects) rCBF would be correlated with severity of the symptom of interest. Partial correlation analysis might be necessary to allow for variance in confounding variables. In some circumstances, a correlational approach within individual subjects is feasible. For example, in attempting to establish the pattern of cerebral activity associated with formal thought disorder, individual subjects with thought disorder might be scanned while generating speech, on multiple occasions, and the correlation between rCBF and the amount of thought disorder during each scan determined.

Cerebral activity associated with task performance

If the object is to establish the pattern of cerebral activity associated with a specific cognitive task that is believed to be implicated in the pathophysiology of schizophrenia, such as internal generation of words, the categorical approach would entail comparing rCBF during the articulation of a list of words generated internally by the subject with rCBF during the articulation of a list of words provided by the experimenter. The interpretation of studies of cerebral activity associated with a specific cognitive task is fraught with difficulty because of the issue of potential variability in the degree of involvement in the mental process of interest. For example, the change in rCBF at a particular cerebral site in schizophrenic patients during performance of a task which the patients have difficulty in performing might be different from that in normal control subjects simply because the patients are less engaged in the task.

In principle, a correlational approach might be used also to identify the cerebral sites involved in a particular aspect of cognitive processing, if it is possible to scan during a series of mental states which involve the relevant aspect of cognitive processing to varying (but quantifiable) degrees. However, it should be noted that evidence from the study of normal subjects during the processing of heard words indicates that, while primary auditory cortex is activated approximately in proportion to the rate of word presentation, auditory association cortical areas tend to be engaged in an all-or-none manner[2]. Thus, caution should be exercised in planning correlational approaches based on the assumption of a linearly increasing activation of a given cerebral area as rate of processing increases, when the object is to explore the function of association cortex. None the less, the correlational approach has proven valuable in establishing those brain areas in which activity increases in proportion to processing load during word list learning in normal individuals[3]. In particular, hippocampal activity was found to be correlated with the amount of processing by the long-term verbal memory system.

Confounding variance in functional images

In addition to the variance arising from differences between or within individuals in current mental activity, there are other sources of systematic variance between images are that less likely to be informative about patterns of brain function, but must be allowed for if the images are to be interpreted correctly. Two of the most important sources of potentially confounding variance are variations over time and between subjects in global cerebral flow or metabolism, and variations between subjects in brain orientation, size and shape.

Variance in global rCBF or rCMRglu

Various systemic metabolic factors such as arterial carbon dioxide level, and perhaps even diurnal variations in hormonal levels, would be expected to alter cerebral blood flow and metabolism, independently of the degree of local neuronal activity. In general, the magnitude of variations in rCBF at a specific cerebral site arising from fluctuations in global flow are as great in magnitude as the variations due to local neural activity. However, a study of the changes in rCBF in the area of motor cortex engaged during voluntary respiration measured at differing levels of arterial carbon dioxide demonstrated that it is possible to treat local rCBF as the sum of two independent contributions: a contribution attributable to local neural activity and a contribution from fluctuations in global flow due to variations in systemic metabolic factors[4]. This indicates that the appropriate way to allow for variance in global flow is analysis of covariance treating global flow as a covariate[5]. That is, examining the relationship between the variable of interest and change in rCBF in each pixel, after removing the effects of variation in global flow on rCBF by linear regression.

Some investigators allow for variation in global flow by a normalization procedure that entails dividing local CBF by global CBF. Such a procedure would only be valid if changes in rCBF due to local neural activity were proportional to global CBF, which is unlikely to be the case. However, the errors anticipated from such a normalization procedure are likely to be small under most circumstances.

Variations in brain structure

Individual variations in brain structure present two related problems for the interpretation of functional imaging studies. The first is variation in the magnitude of the partial volume effect due to variation between subjects in the proportion of grey and white matter in a specific pixel. White matter CBF is lower than grey matter CBF. A lower observed CBF in a specific pixel might reflect lesser activity in the neurones that are present in the pixel or fewer neurones in the pixel.

The second problem is variation between subjects in the location of the neurones which perform a specific task in relation to identifiable structural landmarks. In studies of single subjects, the most appropriate way to illustrate the location of a particular region of activation is to superimpose the functional image on a structural image obtained using MRI. In the case of studies of groups of subjects, it is possible to derive a standard template by superimposing and averaging the MRI images of all group members, and then to determine the plastic transformation required to map the functional image of each individual on to the averaged structural image in a way that produces the best fit according to a least mean square criterion. While this procedure might produce optimal matching with the standard structural template, it would be expected that differences between subjects in the locations of neurones performing a specific aspect of mental processing would remain. Because of this issue of variation in location of the relevant neurones, some investigators have argued that it is preferable simply to perform a plastic transformation that matches the individual's functional image to a standard functional image template derived by averaging a large number of functional images[6].

Cerebral activity associated with expression of symptoms

In general, resting state cerebral activity might be expected to reflect mental state at the time of scanning, and hence functional imaging studies comparing resting state rCBF or rCMRglu in patients with that in controls might be expected to reveal patterns of cerebral activity associated with symptom expression. The first such study was reported by Ingvar and Franzén in 1974[7]. They measured regional cortical blood flow using the xenon infusion technique, in a group of chronic schizophrenic patients, and found relative underactivity of the frontal cortex. They observed that the hypofrontality was related to severity of symptoms such as catatonic underactivity. In the following two decades there was an active debate about whether hypofrontality was a feature of schizophrenia in general or only a feature of chronic patients with slowed psychomotor activity.

Many subsequent functional imaging studies comparing schizophrenic patients with normal controls were performed but the results were conflicting, probably because most of these studies did not pay attention to the issue of the mental state of the subjects at the time of scanning, nor to other sources of confounding variance in the images. Of the 35 studies of resting state rCBF or rCMRglu published in the period 1976 to 1990, 18 reported hypofrontality[8].

The first functional imaging study that made a reasonable attempt to account for the diverse sources of image variance was the PET study of resting rate rCBF in unmedicated schizophrenic patients, in comparison with normal control subjects, by Early and colleagues[9]. They allowed for global variance in rCBF by dividing regional CBF by global CBF, and addressed the issue of variance in brain structure and orientation by using anatomical landmarks to realign the functional images to coincide with a standard template. They found that these acutely ill, unmedicated patients had significantly greater rCBF in the left globus pallidus. There was no evidence of hypofrontality, confirming that the hypofrontality is unlikely to be a general feature of schizophrenia, but more likely to be a feature of the specific mental state of the patients studied by Ingvar and Franzén.

Overall, the evidence from the studies of the first two decades of functional imaging in schizophrenia indicated that there is no single pattern of cerebral activity characteristic of schizophrenia, but suggested that the pattern of cerebral activity varies with the phase of illness, and perhaps with specific symptom profile. To address the issue of the relationship between symptom profile and pattern of cerebral activity, Liddle and colleagues at Hammersmith Hospital, London, carried out a PET study using a between-subject correlation design to measure the correlation between resting state rCBF and symptom severity in a group of medicated patients with persistent stable symptoms[10]. They measured the correlation between rCBF and each of three orthogonal syndromes: psychomotor poverty (poverty of speech; flat affect; decreased spontaneous movement); disorganization (disorders of the form of thought; inappropriate affect); and reality distortion (delusions; hallucinations). Because these syndromes are orthogonal, the correlation between rCBF in a particular pixel and the severity of any one of three syndromes is unlikely to be substantially influenced by variation in severity of either of the other two syndromes. By studying patients with persistent stable symptoms, they maximized the likelihood that the mental state of each patient during scanning would reflect the specific profile of symptoms characteristic of that patient. Analysis of covariance was employed to remove the influence of fluctuation in global blood flow, and a plastic spatial transformation was carried out to match each image with a standard template.

This analysis revealed that psychomotor poverty was associated with decreased rBCF in prefrontal cortex and left parietal cortex, and with increases in rCBF in the caudate nuclei. Disorganization was associated with decreased rCBF in right ventral prefrontal cortex and contiguous insula, and increased rCBF in the right anterior cingulate and in the thalamus. Reality distortion was associated with increased rCBF in the left medial temporal lobe and left lateral prefrontal cortex, and with decreased rCBF in the posterior cingulate, ventral striatum, left superior temporal gyrus and adjacent parietal cortex. Thus, each syndrome was associated with a distributed pattern of cerebral activity in association cortex and related subcortical nuclei.

Furthermore, in the case of each syndrome, the cerebral sites involved included the site maximally activated in normal individuals when performing the type of mental processing which previous neuropsychological studies had shown to be implicated in that syndrome[11]. For example, psychomotor poverty is associated with poor performance in word generation tasks. During such tasks, the area maximally activated in normal individuals[12] coincides with the area of left lateral prefrontal cortex in which there is a negative correlation between psychomotor poverty and rCBF.

In the case of the disorganization syndrome, which involves impaired ability to suppress inappropriate responses, the observed deficit in ventral prefrontal cortex activity is consistent with the evidence that ventral prefrontal lesions in animals produce an impaired ability to suppress inappropriate responses, while the abnormal excess of activity in the anterior cingulate cortex is consistent with the finding that this is the area maximally activated in normal individuals performing the Stroop task[13], a task which patients with marked disorganization perform poorly.

The neuropsychological correlates of the reality distortion syndrome remain in doubt, but some evidence supports the hypothesis that the cardinal deficit is impaired internal monitoring of self-generated mental activity[14]. In a PET study of cerebral activity in normal individuals during the learning of a novel eye-movement task designed to place heavy demands on internal monitoring, one of the cerebral sites strongly activated was the parahippocampal gyrus[14], corresponding to the site at which rCBF is correlated with reality distortion, supporting the hypothesis that reality distortion entails a pathological excess in internal monitoring of self-generated mental activity.

Subsequently, Ebmeier and colleagues[15] used SPET with ^{99m}Tc-HMPAO to measure rCBF in a group of unmedicated, acutely ill patients. They replicated the findings of a negative correlation between psychomotor poverty and left frontal rCBF; the positive correlation between disorganization and rCBF in the right anterior cingulate cortex; and the negative correlation between reality distortion and left lateral temporal rCBF, previously reported by the Hammersmith group. However, they did not find evidence of a positive correlation between reality distortion and left medial temporal flow. The question of whether this discrepancy between the findings of the Hammersmith group and Ebmeier et al arises from the limited sensitivity of SPET to deep brain structures, or from some other unexplained confounding source of variance in one of the two studies, remains unanswered.

Paradoxically, Ebmeier at al found that prefrontal rCBF was greater in the schizophrenic group as a whole than in normal control subjects, despite finding a negative correlation between psychomotor poverty and prefrontal rCBF. This implies that some other aspect of the illness that was prominent in that patient sample, most likely psychomotor excitation, is associated with increased frontal activity.

Other SPET studies have confirmed the relationship between negative symptoms, similar to the symptoms of the psychomotor poverty syndrome, and decreased prefrontal rCBF[16], while PET studies have confirmed the relationship between similar symptoms and decreased rCMRglu[17,18]. Thus, the observation of a negative correlation between psychomotor poverty and prefrontal cerebral activity has proven to be quite robust. However, psychomotor poverty is associated not only with hypofrontality but with a pattern of disturbed cerebral activity in other association cortical areas intimately linked with prefrontal cortex, such as the angular gyrus of the parietal lobe, and in subcortical nuclei[10]. Furthermore, while the cerebral activity is decreased in the cortical areas implicated, it is increased in the subcortical areas. Therefore, it appears that the pattern reflects a state of dynamic imbalance between reciprocally connected brain areas, rather than a fixed loss of function. In the case of each of the other syndromes, the patterns of cerebral activity also appears to reflect dynamic imbalance within a distributed network embracing multimodal association cortex and related subcortical nuclei.

McGuire et al[19] performed a within-subject, categorical study design with SPET to compare rCBF in the presence and absence of auditory hallucinations. They found that auditory hallucinations were associated with increased rCBF in Broca's area, medial prefrontal cortex and medial temporal lobe. It is likely that the increased rCBF in Broca's area reflects cerebral activity specific to the generation of auditory hallucinations in particular, while the increased rCBF in the medial temporal lobe is characteristic of the expression of symptoms of the reality distortion syndrome in general.

Cognitive activation in schizophrenia

The seminal cognitive activation studies in schizophrenia were those performed by Weinberger and colleagues[20] at the National Institute of Mental Health (NIMH) in Washington. They used the xenon inhalation technique to measure regional cortical perfusion during performance of the Wisconsin Card Sorting Test (WCST), a task which demands flexibility of thinking and hence would be expected to engage frontal cortex, compared with a control condition not expected to entail activity of the frontal cortex. They found that schizophrenic patients produced a lesser degree of activation of prefrontal cortex during this task than normal individuals. This finding has subsequently been replicated by the NIMH group[21] and other groups[22]. The degree of prefrontal activation is correlated with the level of the dopaminergic metabolite, homovanillic acid, in the cerebrospinal fluid in schizophrenic patients, implying that the diminished ability to activate prefrontal cortex is related to dopaminergic underactivity[21].

Furthermore, in a study of twins discordant for schizophrenia, the NIMH group[23] found that, in all twin pairs, the affected twin exhibited the lesser degree of prefrontal activation, even in those instances where both twins exhibited a degree of activation within the normal range suggesting that, in all cases of schizophrenia, the ability to activate prefrontal cortex is diminished from what it might have been in the absence of schizophrenia. In the concordant twin pairs, the degree of diminished ability to activate prefrontal cortex did not show any tendency to be greater in the twin with the greater lifetime treatment with medication, confirming that the deficit does not appear to be a consequence of antipsychotic treatment.

While neuropsychological activation studies yield information about cerebral activity associated with the relevant neuropsychological task, rather than providing a direct image of the cerebral activity associated with expression of symptoms, it might, none the less, be anticipated that diminished ability to activate frontal cortex during a frontal task would be correlated with the severity of psychomotor poverty symptoms (core negative symptoms). The NIMH group have not reported such an association. However, in a SPET study of frontal activity during the Tower of London test, a planning task also expected to engage prefrontal cortex, Andreasen et al found that unmedicated schizophrenic patients exhibited lesser activation of medial prefrontal cortex than normal controls and, furthermore, that the degree of diminution of medial frontal activation was correlated with the severity of negative symptoms[8].

The major uncertainty in the interpretation of the findings of diminished frontal activation in schizophrenic patients during performance of frontal tasks such as the WCST and the Tower of London arises from the fact that the schizophrenic patients tend to perform poorly. It is possible that the deficit reflects decreased level of engagement in the task of solving the problem presented. Indeed, in the first NIMH study of cerebral activity during the WCST[20], there was a strong correlation between level of performance achieved and degree of prefrontal activation, though this correlation was not found to be significant in later studies. The possibility of lesser engagement in the specific aspect of the task which is of interest, raises the question of whether or not schizophrenic patients do achieve the same level of prefrontal activation when they perform at the same level as normal individuals.

To address this issue, the Hammersmith group used PET to measure the changes in rCBF in chronic schizophrenic patients during the generation of words at a paced rate of one word every 5 seconds, compared with rCBF during a baseline task in which the patients articulated words provided by the experimenter, at the same rate[24]. In normal individuals, internal generation of words under these circumstances produces a very similar pattern to that seen during unpaced word generation. In particular, normal subjects exhibit an increase in rCBF in left lateral and medial prefrontal cortex and thalamus, and a decrease in rCBF in the lateral temporal lobe. In the schizophrenic patients, paced generation of words was associated with activation of frontal cortex of equal amplitude to that seen in normal subjects performing at the same rate. However, in the schizophrenic patients, the frontal activation tended to be more extensive. In addition, the schizophrenic patients did not produce the normal suppression of activity in left temporal lobe, but actually exhibited an activation in that region. In addition, there was an abnormal activation of parietal cortex, and abnormally extensive suppression of activity in posterior cingulate cortex and the adjacent precuneus.

Thus, the schizophrenic patients were capable of activating prefrontal cortex if paced so as to achieve a rate of word generation comparable with that in normal subjects. However, the pattern of cerebral activity in other areas of multimodal association cortex connected to prefrontal cortex was different in the patients from that in the normal individuals. This altered relationship between frontal cortex and other association cortical areas cannot be ascribed merely to a generalized increase in extent of cortical activation (perhaps associated with greater stress) because the schizophrenic patients showed an abnormal decrease in rCBF in the posterior cingulate cortex and precuneus.

Functional connectivity

The evidence from the studies of rCBF patterns associated with expression of schizophrenic symptoms, and from study of cerebral activation during word generation suggests that the abnormalities of cortical function in schizophrenia comprise a dynamic imbalance between cerebral regions rather than a fixed loss of function. In other words, the abnormalities appear to reflect a disturbance of functional connectivity between cerebral areas. The degree of functional connectivity between two cerebral sites during the performance of specific type of mental process is measured by the correlation between the variation in cerebral activity at the two sites as the degree of engagement in the relevant activity varies.

Ideally, functional connectivity should be measured by repeated measurements in the same individual in a variety of brain states that entail variation in engagement in the relevant mental process. PET rCBF techniques using ^{15}O are suitable for this purpose because it is feasible to perform up to 12 scans in different brain states during a single imaging session. Each image embraces the majority of the brain volume, allowing the measurement of distributed patterns of connectivity. The principal limitations of PET for measuring functional connectivity are the necessary 10-minute interval between scans (while radiation from the previous scan decays to negligible levels), and the fact that the need to limit radiation exposure restricts the total number of allowable scans of each individual. Fast MRI functional imaging techniques are not limited by radiation exposure, and hence have even greater potential for the measurement of functional connectivity, but present techniques do not readily allow imaging of the entire brain.

It is essential to take account of the fact that the degree of functional connectivity between cerebral sites depends on the specific task being performed and, hence, in designing studies of connectivity, it is necessary to choose an appropriate task. For the exploration of disturbances of connectivity in schizophrenia, word generation tasks are likely to be informative. Not only do disturbances of language provide a prominent clinical feature of schizophrenia but also word generation tasks activate a distributed pattern of brain regions including association cortical areas of frontal, temporal and parietal cortex, and related subcortical nuclei, that are implicated in schizophrenia.

Principal component analysis

As brain function can be most accurately described in terms of distributed networks, the most useful approach to describing functional connectivity entails measurement and interpretation of the pairwise correlations between cerebral activity in an extensive network of cerebral sites. If rCBF is measured in an array of pixels of dimensions in the range 2–4 mm, the distributed volume of brain engaged in a task such as word generation spans a set of several thousand pixels. Hence, the covariance matrix that represents the pairwise correlations between rCBF in all the potentially relevant pixels is very large. Interpretation of this extensive set of correlations is difficult unless some form of data reduction is employed to condense the important information into a smaller number of variables. One approach is principal component analysis. Principle component analysis seeks to identify a small number of independent patterns of cerebral activity that account for a large proportion of the covariance between pixels. Each principal component comprises a set of loadings on each of the pixels in the extensive volume of brain engaged in the task.

In the case of normal individuals performing a series of tasks that entail word generation to varying degrees, the first principal component has large positive loadings on pixels in the left lateral and medial prefrontal cortex and thalamus, and negative loadings on pixels in the left superior temporal gyrus[25]. This pattern closely resembles the pattern of difference in rCBF between articulation of a list of words generated internally by the subjects and that during articulation of a list of words provided by the experimenter, and thus appears to reflect the pattern of cerebral activity associated with internal generation of words. In schizophrenic patients, the loadings on the first principal component of the matrix describing the covariance between pixels during the same series of word generation of tasks are substantially different from those seen in normal individuals, implying a different pattern of functional connectivity[26].

Use of the two-norm to quantify patterns of cerebral connectivity

The degree to which the pattern of cerebral connectivity occurring in an individual resembles that occurring in a group of reference subjects can be quantified by use of matrix algebra. Multiplication of the vector representing the first principal component of rCBF accounting for the covariance between pixels during a series of scans in the reference subjects by the matrix representing the pattern of rCBF in the index subject scanned in a similar manner yields a vector whose length is a measure of the overlap between the principal component and the rCBF pattern of the index subject.

The length of a vector is known as its two-norm. The value of the relevant two-norm represents, in simple numerical form, the degree to which a particular individual manifests the pattern of cerebral connectivity occurring in the reference group.

Friston et al[26] calculated the square of the two-norm measuring the degree to which schizophrenic subjects exhibited the pattern of cerebral activity represented by the first principal component of rCBF for a group of normal subjects scanned while generating words. They found that, in the schizophrenic patients, the mean value of this measure of the extent of occurrence of the normal pattern of cerebral activity was only one-twentieth of the value expected for a normal individual. This indicates that schizophrenic patients exhibit a substantially different pattern of functional connectivity during word generation.

Pharmacological challenge studies

PET measurements of rCBF can be employed to study the effect of pharmacological agents on cerebral function. Depending on the type of information sought, rCBF can be imaged before and after a single dose of a pharmacological agent, or before and after a sustained period of treatment. When studying the effects of pharmacological agents acting on monoaminergic systems, it is necessary to be cautious about interpretation of changes in rCBF since monoaminergic agents are prone to exhibit direct vasoactive effects. For measurement of sustained effects of pharmacological agents, it is probably preferable to measure regional glucose metabolism using ^{18}F-deoxyglucose. For measurement of the acute effects of a pharmacological agent on a particular type of mental processing, rCBF techniques are preferable, because they allow multiple repeated scans. If the object is to measure the effect of a pharmacological agent on the difference in rCBF between a mental state of interest and a control mental state, direct vasoactive effects unrelated to local neural activity would not confound the measurement provided they are similar in the test condition and in the control condition.

An illustration of the single dose challenge strategy is provided by the PET study examining the effects of the dopamine agonist apomorphine on regional glucose metabolism in normal individuals and in schizophrenic patients, performed by Cleghorn et al[27]. Apomorphine produced a decrease in metabolism in the corpus striatum in schizophrenic subjects, but did not change striatal metabolism significantly in normal controls. This observation is consistent with evidence from several studies using PET to measure glucose metabolism before and after treatment[28,29], indicating that sustained dopaminergic blockade can increase striatal metabolism in at least some schizophrenic patients. Buchsbaum et al[29] found that the effect that sustained dopaminergic blockade with haloperidol on striatal metabolism was related to treatment responsivity. Patients who responded well to treatment with haloperidol had an abnormally low striatal metabolism while taking placebo, and exhibited a significant increase in striatal metabolism during treatment.

In view of the fact that monoamine neurotransmitters such as dopamine act as neuromodulators which regulate the tone of the concurrent brain activity, perhaps the most informative strategy for investigating the effects of dopaminergic agonists or antagonists is to measure the effects they have on the patterns of cerebral activity associated with specific mental processes. Such a strategy entails the combination of neuropharmacological with neuropsychological challenge. The first studies of this type were performed by the NIMH group using the xenon inhalation technique to examine the effect of the indirect dopaminergic agonist, amphetamine, on the prefrontal rCBF during the Wisconsin Card Sorting Test. They found that amphetamine tended to alleviate the deficit in prefrontal activation during the WCST in the schizophrenic patients and, furthermore, produced a slight alleviation of the WCST performance deficit[30].

Although the findings from pharmacological activation studies must be interpreted with caution until the validity and reliabilty of the techniques have been confirmed by more extensive application, the studies that have imaged glucose metabolism or rCBF during pharmacological challenge, either alone or in combination with neuropsychological challenge, suggest that dopaminergic agonists decrease striatal metabolism in schizophrenic patients (but not in normal individuals) while at least partially alleviating the deficit in ability to activate the prefrontal cortex. Overall, this preliminary evidence from pharmacological challenge studies supports the hypothesis that the pathophysiology of schizophrenia entails underactivity of prefrontal dopaminergic projections and hyperactivity of subcortical dopaminergic projections.

Conclusions

PET studies reveal a complex pattern of cerebral dysfunction in schizophrenia. The expression of each of the three major classes of characteristic schizophrenic symptoms is associated with a different pattern of cerebral activity in multimodal association cortical areas[10]. Furthermore, many studies[8,20–23] have demonstrated that schizophrenic patients have an impaired ability to activate prefrontal cortex during frontal lobe tasks. However, when performance in a word generation task is paced so that schizophrenic patients produce words at the same rate as normal controls, the magnitude of prefrontal activation in the schizophrenic subjects is similar to that in the normals[24]. Under these circumstances, the abnormality lies in the functional connectivity between frontal lobes and other multimodal association cortical areas. This description of schizophrenia as a disorder of functional connectivity between cerebral areas provides a parallel to Bleuler's description of schizophrenia in psychological terms as a disorder of the associations within and between different mental activities; a fragmentation of the mind which led him to name the illness schizophrenia.

References

(1) Neil JJ. Functional imaging of the central nervous system using magnetic resonance imaging and positron emission tomography. *Curr Opin Neurol Neurosurg* 1993; 6: 927–33.

(2) Price C, Wise R, Ramsay S et al. Regional response differences within the human auditory cortex when listening to words. *Neurosci Lett* 1992; 146: 179–82.

(3) Grasby PM, Frith CD, Friston KJ, Frackowiak RSJ, Dolan RJ. Activation of the human hippocampal formation during auditory–verbal long-term memory function. *Neurosci Lett* 1993; 163: 185–8.

(4) Ramsay SC, Murphy K, Shea SA et al. Changes in global cerebral blood flow in humans: effects on regional cerebral blood flow during a neural activation task. *J Physiol (Lond)* 1993; 471: 521–34.

(5) Friston KJ, Frith CD, Liddle PF, Lammertsma AA, Dolan RD, Frackowiak RSJ. The relationship between global and local changes in PET scans. *J Cereb Blood Flow Metab* 1990; 10: 458–66.

(6) Friston KJ, Frith CD, Liddle PF, Frackowiak RSJ. Plastic transformation of PET images. *J Comput Ass Tomog* 1991; 15: 634–9.

(7) Ingvar DH, Franzén G. Abnormalities of cerebral blood flow distribution in patients with chronic schizophrenia. *Acta Psychiat Scand* 1974; 50: 425–62.

(8) Andreasen NC, Rezai K, Alliger R et al. Hypofrontality in neuroleptic–naive patients and in patients with chronic schizophrenia. Assessment with xenon 133 single-photon emission computed tomography and the Tower of London. *Arch Gen Psychiat* 192; 49: 943–58.

(9) Early TS, Reiman ER, Raichle ME, Spitznagel EL. Left globus pallidus abnormality in never-medicated patients with schizophrenia. *Proc Natl Acad Sci USA* 1987; 84: 561–3.

(10) Liddle PF, Friston KJ, Frith CD, Jones T, Hirsch SR, Frackowiak RSJ. Patterns of cerebral blood flow in schizophrenia. *Br J Psychiat* 1992; 160: 179–86.

(11) Liddle PF, Friston KJ, Frith CD, Frackowiak RSJ. Cerebral blood flow and mental processes in schizophrenia. *J Roy Soc Med* 1992; 85: 224–7.

(12) Frith CD, Friston KJ, Liddle PF, Frackowiak RSJ. Willed action and the prefrontal cortex in man: a study with PET. *Proc Roy Soc (Lond) B* 1991; 24: 241–6.

(13) Pardo JV, Pardo PJ, Janer KW, Raichle ME. The anterior cingulate mediates processing selection in the Stroop attentional conflict paradigm. *Proc Natl Acad Sci USA* 1990; 87: 256–9.

(14) Frith CD, Friston KJ, Liddle PF, Frackowiak RSJ. PET imaging and cognition in schizophrenia. *J Roy Soc Med* 1992; 85: 222–4.

(15) Ebmeier KP, Blackwood DHR, Murray C et al. Single photon emission tomography with ^{99m}Tc-exametazime in unmedicated schizophrenic patients. *Biol Psychiat* 1993; 33: 487–95.
(16) Suzuki M, Kurachi M, Kawasaki Y, Kiba K, Yamaguchi N. Left hypofrontality correlates with blunted affect in schizophrenia. *Jpn J Psychiat Neurol* 1992; 46: 653–7.
(17) Wolkin A, Sanfilipo M, Wolf AP, Angrist B, Brodie JD, Rotrosen J. Negative symptoms and hypofrontality in chronic schizophrenia. *Arch Gen Psychiat* 1992; 49: 959–65.
(18) Tamminga CA, Thaker GK, Buchanan R et al. Limbic system abnormalities identified in schizophrenia using positron emission tomography with fluorodeoxyglucose and neocortical alterations with deficit syndrome. *Arch Gen Psychiat* 1992; 49: 522–30.
(19) McGuire PK, Shah GMS, Murray RM. Increased blood flow in Broca's area during auditory hallucinations in schizophrenia. *Lancet* 1993; 342: 703–6.
(20) Weinberger DR, Berman KF, Zec RF. Physiologic dysfunction of dorsolateral prefrontal cortex in schizophrenia. 1. Regional cerebral blood flow evidence. *Arch Gen Psychiat* 1986; 43: 114–24.
(21) Weinberger DR, Berman KF, Illowsky BP. Physiological dysfunction of the dorsolateral prefrontal cortex in schizophrenia. III. A new cohort and evidence for a monoaminergic mechanism. *Arch Gen Psychiat* 1988; 45: 609–15.
(22) Rubin P, Holm S, Friberg L et al. Altered modulation of prefrontal and subcortical activity in newly diagnosed schizophrenia and schizophreniform disorder. *Arch Gen Psychiat* 1991; 48: 987–95.
(23) Berman KF, Torrey EF, Daniel DG, Weinberger DR. Regional cerebral blood flow in monozygotic twins discordant and concordant for schizophrenia. *Arch Gen Psychiat* 1992; 49: 927–35.
(24) Liddle PF, Herold S, Fletcher P, Friston KJ, Silbersweig D, Frith CD. A PET study of word generation in schizophrenia. *Schizophrenia Res* 1994; 11: 168.
(25) Friston KJ, Frith CD, Liddle PF, Frackowiak RSJ. Functional connectivity: the principal component analysis of large (PET) data sets. *J Cereb Blood Flow Metab* 1993; 13: 5–14.
(26) Friston KJ, Herold S, Fletcher P et al. Abnormal fronto–temporal interaction in schizophrenia. In: Watson SJ, ed. *Biology of schizophrenia and affective disorders.* New York: Raven Press; 1994.
(27) Cleghorn JM, Szechtman H, Garnett E et al. Apomorphine effects on brain metabolism in neuroleptic–naive schizophrenic patients. *Psychiat Res: Neuroimaging* 1991; 40: 135–53.
(28) Szechtman H, Nahmias C, Garnett ES et al. Effects of neuroleptics on altered cerebral glucose metabolism in schizophrenia. *Arch Gen Psychiat* 1988; 45: 523–32.
(29) Buchsbaum MS, Potkin SG, Sigel BV et al. Striatal metabolic rate and clinical response to neuroleptics in schizophrenia. *Arch Gen Psychiat* 1992; 49: 966–74.
(30) Daniel DG, Weinberger DR, Jones DW et al. The effect of amphetamine on regional cerebral blood flow during cognitive activation in schizophrenia. *J Neurosci* 1991; 11: 1907–17.

In vitro brain imaging: techniques for studying and localizing the pathogenesis of psychiatric diseases

P J HARRISON

Introduction

The ideal neuroimaging machine would have many characteristics. It would have the ability to measure any desired parameter of brain structure or function in vivo, in a way which was entirely specific and accurate in molecular and spatial terms. It would be non-invasive, safe, rapid, reliable and unaffected by short-term state variables.

The contributions in this volume illustrate the rapid strides being made by neuroimaging towards these goals, and the consequent advances in neurobiological understanding of psychiatric diseases which are occurring. However, it also remains true that the ideals are not yet attainable. For many research purposes there continues to be no substitute for the direct examination of brain tissue. Fortunately, the extraordinary advances of molecular biology, which eclipse even those of neuroimaging, have greatly increased the power and value of traditional post-mortem studies. This chapter discusses some methods in the latter category from the standpoint that they represent in vitro counterparts of in vivo imaging.

As a rule, molecular biological methods are highly specific and sensitive, whilst the imaging component allows studies to occur at an accurate spatial resolution. These properties are all essential, given that the neuropathological substrates of brain diseases are in the main highly selective in both molecular and anatomical terms. The technique which currently best demonstrates the combination of molecular specificity with anatomical detail is in situ hybridization histochemistry (ISHH)[1–4]. Here, the principles of ISHH and examples of its applications to psychiatric disorders are outlined. Related techniques are also discussed.

All correspondence to: Dr P J Harrison, University Department of Psychiatry, Warneford Hospital, Oxford OX3 7JX, UK.

Cambridge Medical Reviews: Neurobiology and Psychiatry Volume 3

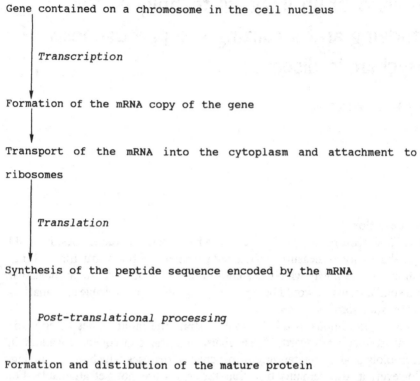

Gene contained on a chromosome in the cell nucleus

↓ *Transcription*

Formation of the mRNA copy of the gene

↓

Transport of the mRNA into the cytoplasm and attachment to ribosomes

↓ *Translation*

Synthesis of the peptide sequence encoded by the mRNA

↓ *Post-translational processing*

Formation and distibution of the mature protein

Fig. 1. A simplified flow diagram of the gene expression pathway. The main processes are shown in italics: *transcription*, whereby a faithful mRNA copy is made of the gene, and *translation*, by which the mRNA acts as a template and whose sequence determines the aminoacid sequence of the protein to be made. *Post-translational processing* encompasses the many ways in which the protein is modified before it is functionally complete; for example, it may be glycosylated, phosphorylated or cleaved.

In vitro imaging: in situ hybridization histochemistry (ISHH)

ISHH is a tool for the study of gene expression because it allows messenger RNA (mRNA) to be detected. Messenger RNA is of interest because it is the key intermediate on the gene expression pathway. Each gene gives rise to a different mRNA, which forms the template upon which synthesis of the encoded protein occurs (Fig. 1). A given mRNA is only made by a cell when the protein is being made; thus, finding an mRNA present tells you that the gene is being expressed[5].

Like other related hybridization methods, ISHH relies on the fact that a length of DNA or RNA (the 'probe') will, under suitable conditions, bind ('hybridize') to a strand of DNA or RNA which is complementary to it. Complementary in this context refers to the genetic code: the four nucleotides making up the genetic alphabet, denoted A, C, G and T/U, always pair up between the strands such that A hybridizes to T/U and C hybridizes to G. Thus, for example, a probe with sequence ACGGTC will hybridize to a target nucleic acid of sequence TGCCAG. If the probe is labelled with a marker before use, the site and intensity of hybridization can be detected; radioactive labelling followed by autoradiographic detection is usually used, though non-radioactive methods are also available[6,7]. The unique feature of ISHH is that it is carried out on intact sections of tissue, preserving the anatomical detail and relationships between cells. In contrast, traditional 'grind and bind' methods involve homogenization of chunks of brain tissue and loss of this relationship. Anatomical integrity is especially important in the brain where cell populations are differentiated, e.g. into neurones and glia, astrocytes and oligodendrocytes, pyramidal and Purkinje cells, groups which may be selectively affected by a disease. Images can be produced either by placing the hybridized section against radiosensitive film to show the regional distribution of an mRNA (Fig. 2), or can be studied at the cellular level by dipping the section in liquid emulsion and visualizing grains over individuals neurones (Fig. 3).

ISHH is in many ways similar to immunocytochemistry (ICC), except that ICC detects a protein whilst ISHH detects an mRNA[8]. Both techniques allow measurements at the cellular level. Both have advantages and drawbacks and, in practice, the two are complementary, working best in combination. For example, many proteins are distributed throughout the dendrites and/or axon of a neurone. Thus, a diffuse staining pattern with ICC is often seen, which prevents the cell of origin of the protein from being identified and precludes quantitative estimations of how much protein is in the cell (Fig. 4). In contrast, mRNA is usually limited to cell bodies, so the ISHH signal representing the mRNA is restricted to this site. This allows the neurones expressing the gene to be identified with confidence (Fig. 3). Moreover, the strength of hybridization can be measured, e.g. by counting the autoradiographic grains[4,9–11], with increased signal meaning that more mRNA is present and, as a rule, more protein is being made.

The ability to quantify gene expression, in terms of amount of mRNA present, is important, since changes in the rate of gene expression is a primary means by which cells regulate their metabolism in both physiological and pathological states[4,5,12]. Thus, quantitative ISHH studies of mRNA have been widely used to investigate up- and downregulation of gene expression in specific neuronal populations in response to factors such as ageing, pharmacological treatments or Alzheimer's disease (see below).

The specificity of ISHH in practice is usually greater than ICC since ISHH is based on the genetic code, whereas ICC relies on antigen–antibody recognition. In addition, many individual genes give rise to several mRNAs, called isoforms, which differ only slightly and in turn encode proteins which

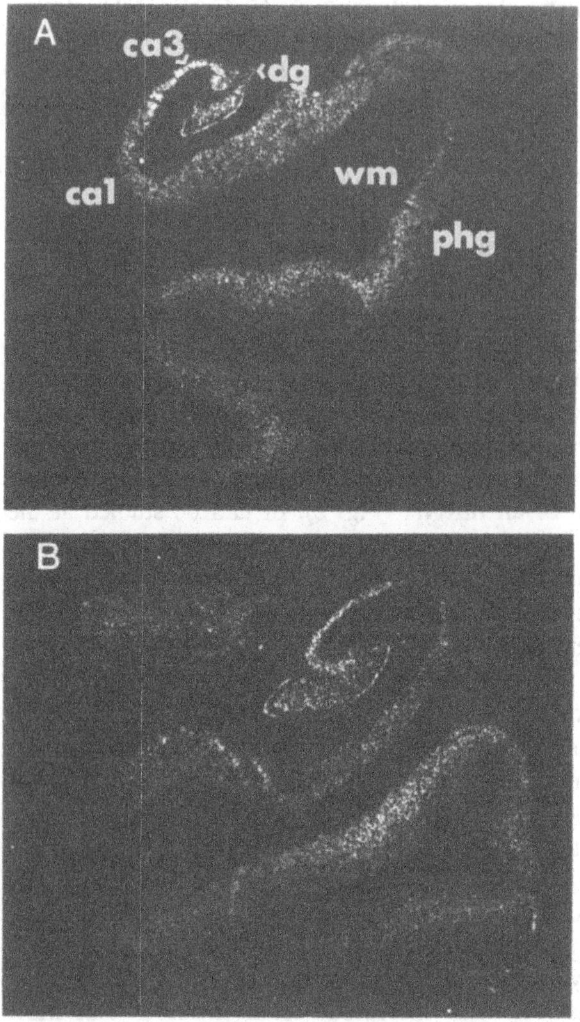

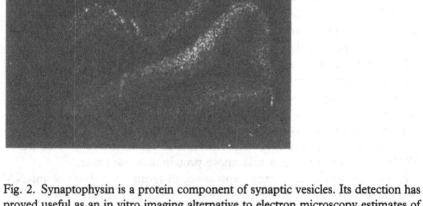

Fig. 2. Synaptophysin is a protein component of synaptic vesicles. Its detection has proved useful as an in vitro imaging alternative to electron microscopy estimates of synaptic density, a parameter of interest in Alzheimer's disease, schizophrenia and other situations[22,90,91]. The distribution of synaptophysin mRNA in the hippocampus of a normal control (A) and a schizophrenic case (B) is shown here after ISHH with a ^{35}S-labelled probe and exposure of the sections to autoradiographic film for three weeks. Increasing whiteness of the image in a given region reflects a combination of the abundance of the mRNA and the density of cells expressing it. Note that no significant synaptophysin mRNA is seen in the white matter (wm), since synaptophysin is only expressed by neurones. eg: dentate gyrus, granule cell layer. ca3, cal: pyramidal neurone fields of Ammon's horn. phg: parahippocampal gyrus.

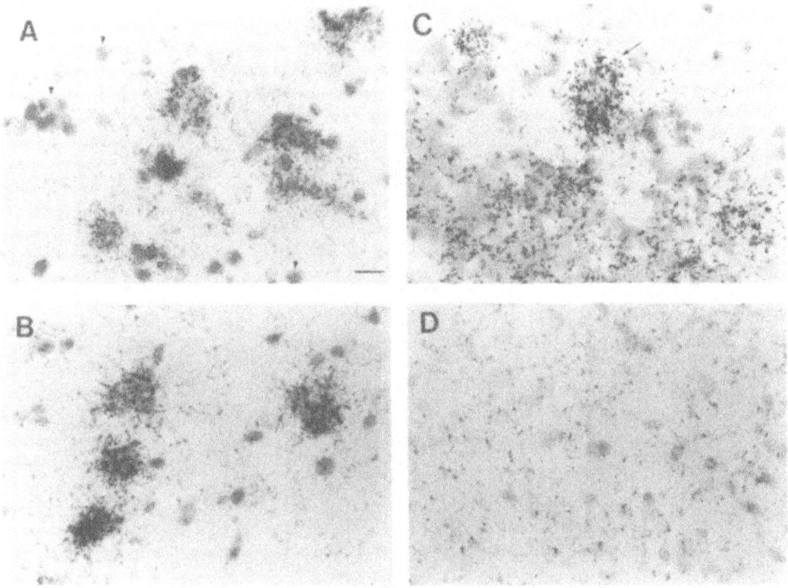

Fig. 3. The distribution of synaptophysin RNA over neurones within the hippocampus (A: CA4 field, B: CA1 field), cerebellum (C) and white matter (D) of postmortem normal human brains. The cell bodies are visualized by counterstaining the section with cresyl violet. The abundance of the mRNA is now represented by the number of grains; cell density is not relevant, unlike in Fig. 2, since the grain count over individual cells can be measured. Synaptophysin mRNA is seen to be expressed primarily by large, pyramidal neurones in hippocampus (A, B) and cerebellar Purkinje cells (arrowed in C). Many of the smaller cells are devoid of grains; these are glia (arrowheads in A) which do not express synaptophysin. D: Absence of significant grains over white matter. Bar: 10 microns.

are also very similar to each other[13,14]. Using appropriately designed probes and experimental conditions, ISHH allows these isoforms to be distinguished, whereas antibodies for ICC may be unable to differentiate reliably between them. This molecular specificity proves to be essential in many situations. For example, glutamate receptors belong to a large gene family[15]. Several of the individual genes are expressed as forms which are molecularly very similar but whose distribution, neurodevelopmental profile and functional characteristics are distinct. ISHH has allowed these isoforms to be differentially mapped[16–18], providing an essential part of the unravelling of their complex properties and potential roles in schizophrenia and other disorders[19,20].

On the other hand, ICC has advantages over ISHH. ICC confirms that the mRNA was indeed being used to make protein, helps show that there

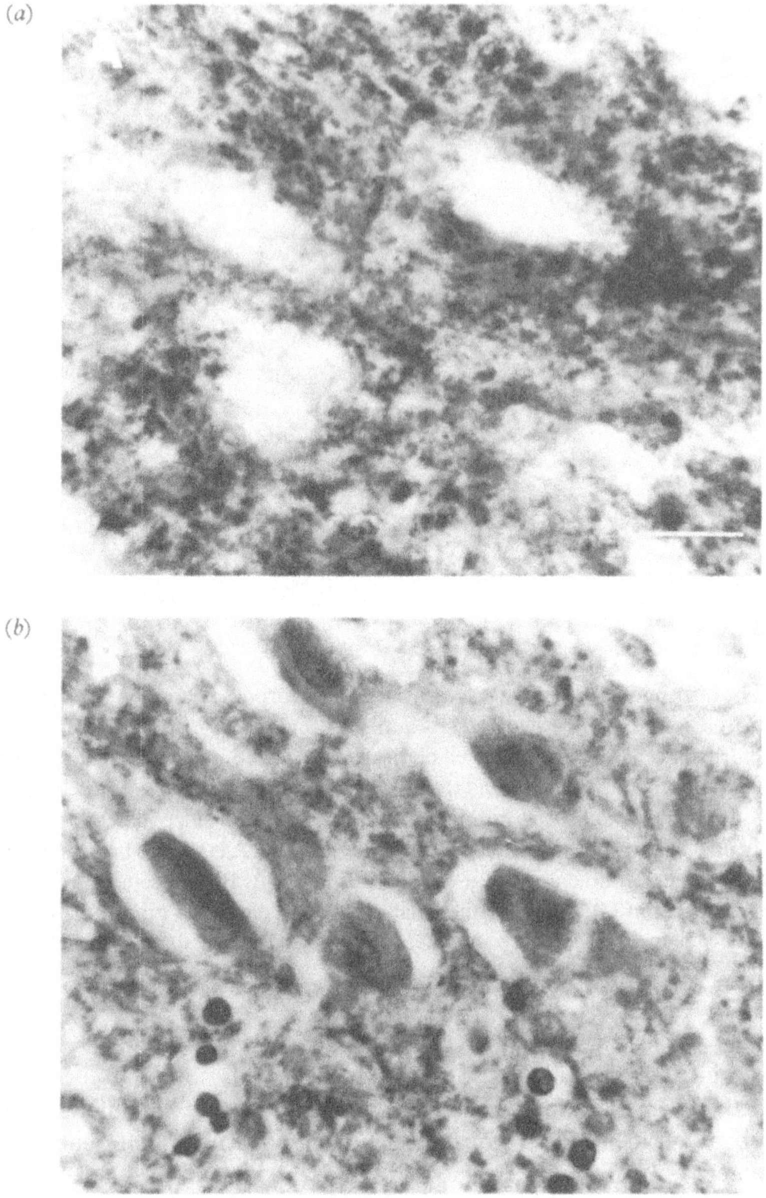

Fig. 4. Synaptophysin detected immunocytochemically in the CA3 field of the hippocampus, using a monoclonal antibody and the avidin–biotin method. (*a*) Neuronal cell bodies are not stained, since synaptophysin is transported to, and concentrated in, the synaptic terminals of neurones. These show up as the dense punctate staining in the surrounding neurophil. (*b*) A similar section, which has been counterstained with cresyl violet to confirm the location of the non-immunoreactive neuronal cell bodies. Bar: 20 microns.

is the predicted relationship between mRNA content and protein abundance[21–23], and tracks where in the cell that protein ended up. There may, for instance, be abnormalities in translation (the process by which the mRNA template is used for protein synthesis) or post-translational processing (the modification of newly produced proteins necessary for their final structure, function and distribution; Fig. 1). Neither of these will be apparent if only the mRNA is studied. For example, the cytoskeletal protein *tau* is the main component of the neurofibrillary tangles which characterize Alzheimer's disease. The primary abnormality of *tau* in Alzheimer's disease seems to be that it undergoes excess and abnormal phosphorylation, even though its expression in terms of distribution of its mRNA is largely, if not entirely, normal[24,25].

Given the complementary roles of ISHH and ICC, methods have been developed to allow both to be carried out on a single section. Thus, both mRNA and protein products of a single gene, or of separate genes whose relationship is of interest[26,27], can be studied simultaneously. In a similar vein, double-labelling techniques allow two mRNAs or two proteins to be concurrently visualized[28,29]. It is also possible to combine ISHH and ICC with methods for tracing neural connections[30]. These approaches illustrate the increasing ability to overcome the 'backwardness' of human neuroanatomy and related disciplines[31]. In general, however, such sophisticated combinations of techniques result in a loss of sensitivity of each component, and this must be weighed against the advantages to be gained.

Apart from ISHH and ICC, the third main in vitro imaging tool feasible in post-mortem human brain tissue is receptor autoradiography[32]. Like ICC, it detects proteins, but relies on ligand binding for its specificity. Like ISHH, detection is carried out by radiolabelling the ligand. It has diminished somewhat in popularity with the emergence of ISHH and ICC, partly because ICC is often more specific for the desired target receptor, and because quantification at the cellular level is easier for technical and conceptual reasons with ISHH[4]. However, it continues to play a useful adjunctive role in many situations, some of which are mentioned below.

Extensions of ISHH and related techniques

ISHH has become a routine tool for the neuroscientist, and its success has led to technical developments to increase the power and range of its applications. The polymerase chain reaction (PCR) allows even single molecules of DNA to be amplified exponentially until the DNA sequence is abundant enough to be detected easily[33]. PCR has been adapted so that mRNA can be similarly copied, overcoming the not infrequent problem that an mRNA is present at levels below the detection threshold of hybridization techniques. This form of PCR involves copying the initial mRNA back into DNA, by the process of reverse transcription, followed by standard PCR (called RT-PCR[26]). There are now techniques by which this process can also be carried out on tissue sections, combining the unequalled detection sensitivity of PCR with some of the anatomical resolution of ISHH[34]. At present these methods are in their infancy, but are likely to become established research tools in the near future.

Other extensions of ISHH take its ability to localize gene expression to the limit. Electron microscopy can be used to identify precisely where the mRNA is present within a neurone[35]; this is useful since the spatial distribution of mRNAs within different cell domains is an important regulator of gene expression[36]. For example, some mRNAs are transported into dendrites[37,38] while in rare instances they are also present in axons[39]. The mRNA profile of individual cells can be studied by inserting a micropipette into a single neurone, aspirating the cytoplasm and performing a modified hybridization in the pipette tip. Additional parameters can also be measured at the same time, allowing correlations between gene expression activity and functional activities of the cell. Such techniques have been used, for example, to investigate whether individual cells in the striatum co-express dopamine receptors, an unresolved issue of importance for understanding basal ganglia circuitry and its involvement in diseases and medication effects[40].

These increasingly arcane-sounding methodologies gain relevance when the nature of the pathology of certain psychiatric conditions is appreciated. Schizophrenia, for example, clearly does not show neuropathological features of a magnitude or overtness seen in the major neurodegenerative disorders; its neurobiological basis is likely to reside at the level of aberrant cytoarchitecture, synaptic organization or the dysfunction of discrete neurone populations[41]. This subtlety of pathology will require equally subtle and powerful experimental techniques for its identification. It is tools such as those outlined here which come into this category.

A separate development, also related to ISHH, is the antisense manipulation of gene expression[42]. Here, a DNA probe which is complementary ('antisense') to an mRNA is infused into the brain of a living animal. It suppresses the translation of the targeted mRNA into its protein and has been used, for example, to downregulate the synthesis of a glutamate receptor[43]. The effects of antisense can be measured behaviourally or pathophysiologically, and can subsequently be confirmed in terms of downregulation of the mRNA or its protein using ISHH, ICC, receptor autoradiography or other neurochemical methods in the brain after death. The antisense approach has both investigative and therapeutic possibilities, and provides a striking fusion of in vivo and in vitro methods[42].

Limitations of in vitro imaging

There are practical and conceptual limitations to in vitro imaging. The quantity and quality of tissue is perhaps the main limitation, a point which emphasizes the importance of resources for systematic collection of brains from patients and suitable controls after death. This is often a neglected aspect of research. It also highlights the need to adapt these techniques to work successfully on routinely processed and archival material[44,45]. Tissue quality in this context includes the adequacy of clinical documentation, whether the cases which come to autopsy are representative of the disease in question and the confounding effects of terminal illnesses and post-mortem interval. With regard to the latter factors, the data indicate that ISHH, ICC, receptor autoradiography and similar techniques are surprisingly resistant to, but are by no means immune from, such confounders, and considerable attention must be paid to controlling for them[22,46–49].

Conceptually, there is always the concern that post-mortem studies can only show a single time point in a given case, and that any group differences or correlations which are observed cannot be assumed to be causally related to any other variable. That is, only associations are detected which in turn allow only weak inferences about their pathobiological significance to be drawn[50]. This is no more or less a problem for in vitro imaging than for other techniques. There are two main ways out of this dilemma. Firstly, by combining post-mortem studies with other experimental approaches and demonstrating congruency of results; for example, possible changes in brain dopamine receptors in schizophrenia can be studied in vivo, using PET or SPECT, and in vitro, using receptor autoradiography or ISHH. Secondly, if there are pre-existing hypotheses which can be critically tested, often in conjunction with appropriate studies in laboratory animals, cell culture or other experimental situations. A recent example of this kind concerns the role of glutamate and the cytoskeleton in the development of schizophrenia[51].

Applications of in vitro imaging

Used in isolation, in vitro imaging is little more than a means by which the molecular endophenotype of the brain can be described in ever more detail. One could continue until the distribution and relative abundance of all 30 000 brain-expressed genes, not to mention all their isoforms, are mapped at both mRNA and protein level throughout the brain. With regard to the neurobiology of psychiatry, however, a more critical application of these techniques is required, in keeping with the need to minimize the conceptual limitations of post-mortem research outlined above. Such uses of in vitro imaging come into four main categories, exemplified here by reference to recent ISHH studies.

Localizing the expression of genes of pathogenic interest

Senile plaques are a characteristic feature of Alzheimer's disease. Once their main constituent had been identified as the β-amyloid peptide, the gene encoding the precursor of this peptide, called the amyloid precursor protein

(APP) gene, became of great interest[52]. From 1987, when the APP gene was sequenced, probes could be designed to allow the expression of the APP gene to be studied in Alzheimer's disease brains. This work provided the first good example of ISHH work directly relevant to psychiatric disorders. It showed clearly that APP is expressed in neurones throughout the brain. Thus, its expression and, by implication, the formation of APP, is a normal event which is not limited to brains or areas of brains affected by Alzheimer's disease. In addition, these data made it unnecessary to propose that the amyloid deposited in diseased brains is synthesized elsewhere in the body and transported via the vasculature, a possibility which had previously been under active consideration.

The molecular picture became complicated after the APP gene was shown to be expressed as three major isoforms which encode APP variants with differing properties. Subsequent ISHH studies therefore investigated these isoforms individually, and showed that one form of APP mRNA is only expressed in neurones, whilst others are expressed in non-neuronal cells too (e.g. glia)[25,51,52]. However, again there seems to be no clear spatial relationship between the distribution of each APP gene product and the pathological features of Alzheimer's disease. Attention therefore turned to the question of whether differences in the *amount* of APP expressed could explain the amyloid pathology of AD (see below).

Many other genes have now had their expression patterns studied in Alzheimer's disease and other brain disorders. There are examples of disease-associated alterations, such as the somatodendritic distribution of the cytoskeletal protein *tau* in Alzheimer's disease neurones[24]. However, changes in localization of mRNAs or proteins seem to be unusual, and it has proved to be differences in the rate or amount of gene expression which are more commonly observed. This emphasizes the value of using in vitro imaging techniques in a quantitative mode.

Quantitative changes in gene expression

In the light of the role of APP in Alzheimer's disease, increased APP expression (in terms of mRNA abundance) has been repeatedly looked for in brains affected by the disease, since it would be a plausible basis for increased amyloid peptide formation and deposition. In the event, in vitro imaging, using quantitative ISHH and related methods to measure levels of APP mRNA, has shown this hypothesis to be false[52]. It was then postulated that there might be changes in the relative abundance of one APP isoform to another, since the encoded APP variants might vary in their propensity to form β-amyloid peptide[53,54]. In several small studies, changes in the ratios of individual APP mRNAs have been found which are localized to different neuronal populations. For example, the amount of one major APP mRNA isoform, called APP695, is increased in some subcortical nuclei[55,56]. In the hippocampus and cortex, the data are conflicting, although ISHH has rarely been used, nor have the studies compared identical cortical regions[52,57]. It is, therefore, possible that localized changes in APP expression might have been missed, especially since ICC data suggest that certain cell groups may contain more APP in Alzheimer's disease than in controls[58]. Studies which have attempted to correlate the expression of APP mRNAs with the local or overall density of senile plaques (as a measure of β-amyloid deposition) have also generally been unsuccessful[6,59,60].

In total, the existing data indicate that abnormalities in the distribution or abundance of APP expression do not play a key role in accounting for the undoubted involvement of this molecule and its derivatives in the pathogenesis of Alzheimer's disease. This conclusion, whilst negative, has played a positive Popperian part in focusing attention on other aspects of APP metabolism which are abnormal in the disease[61,62]. In passing, the recent finding that APP mRNA is affected by mode of death may require some of the previous studies to be reinterpreted or repeated, since this variable has often not been matched between case and control groups[57].

In other situations, in vitro imaging has contributed more directly positive data. Several of these concern non-APP gene products of interest in Alzheimer's disease[44,63,64]. The proposed involvement of glutamate receptors in schizophrenia has already been mentioned. Much of the evidence comes from in vitro imaging which, as with the case of APP in Alzheimer's disease, shows that alterations are both molecularly and spatially complex. In medial temporal lobe, the non-NMDA subtype of glutamate receptor is expressed at reduced levels; this has been shown both by receptor autoradiography and ISHH[65,66]. It remains to be seen which individual members of the non-NMDA receptor gene family account for this overall loss; at the last count there were seven to be studied. Similarly, the fact that a different pattern of glutamatergic involvement is seen in frontal cortex in schizophrenia indicates the need to continue the mapping of these changes as well[67]. As a final example, in Parkinson's disease, cell populations within the substantia nigra show differential changes in mRNAs which may relate to their disease vulnerability[68,69].

The expression of candidate genes

A candidate gene is one which is thought to be centrally involved in the causation of a disease, usually by virtue of a mutation in the gene, or because particular variants (polymorphisms) of the gene are associated with an increased incidence of the disease. In the simplest terms, a gene mutation is pathogenic either because it results in the normal expression of an abnormally functioning protein, or because it results in the abnormal expression of a normally functioning protein. Thus, one important step in bridging the gap between gene mutations and the associated syndrome is to identify where the gene is expressed and to correlate its location and abundance with the clinical and pathological data. This gives in vitro imaging an important role whenever a candidate gene is found or postulated.

Although APP is probably crucial in all forms of Alzheimer's disease[61], it is only in rare forms of familial early-onset disease where APP is unequivocally the cause, by virtue of a gene mutation. The first Alzheimer's disease-causing APP mutation to be discovered[70] was suggested to be pathogenic because it was predicted to alter and stabilize the structure of its encoded mRNA[71], allowing excess APP to be synthesized from it; this in turn provides more substrate for the production of β-amyloid peptide. However, ISHH showed that levels of APP mRNA in the hippocampus and neocortex of this case were no different from controls, making this explanation unlikely[72].

More recently, polymorphisms of the apolipoprotein E gene have been found to be a major determinant of all forms of Alzheimer's disease[73]. In vitro imaging of apolipoprotein E mRNA and protein has already indicated that it is associated with senile plaques[74,75] and is overexpressed in affected brains[76], originating mainly from glia rather than neurones. Such data form part of the attempts to explain why this molecule seems to have a key role in Alzheimer's disease and how it may interact with APP.

The demonstration that Huntington's disease is caused by abnormalities in the IT15 gene[77] does not explain why or how the disease arises in affected individuals, and has therefore been followed by the first studies of IT15 gene expression[78,79]. ISHH and ICC studies of the IT15 gene product will help show, for example, whether its expression pattern explains the strikingly selective vulnerability of discrete neuronal populations to the disease[80].

As a final example, equivalent studies of candidate genes will also be valuable in due course in the psychoses, although the main problem there is to decide which genes are plausible candidates[81,82].

Related experimental studies

Each of the above categories of in vitro imaging are also used in various experimental situations to complement the work in human brains. For example, the expression of APP and apolipoprotein E have been studied in laboratory animals to see what happens after various forms of neural insult or injury[83–87]. One problem with schizophrenia research is to distinguish changes in the brain which are due to the disease from those arising from medication; thus, the expression of many genes has been studied in rats treated with psychotropic drugs to help this distinction[88–90].

Conclusions

In vitro imaging as an experimental approach has been revitalized by the addition of molecular biological techniques to the range of methods which can be carried out on brain tissue. It is now possible to determine accurately the location and abundance of individual gene products, mRNAs as well as proteins, to neurones in sections of brain, using techniques such as ISHH and ICC. Like most imaging approaches, in vitro imaging has its forte in clarifying pathogenic, rather than aetiological, processes. In the case of Alzheimer's disease and several other neurodegenerative disorders, the use of these methods in harness with other molecular genetic techniques has already led to fundamental breakthroughs. In schizophrenia, the advances are at an earlier stage, but they are contributing to the renaissance of neurobiological research into the disease. The data indicate that in vitro imaging will remain one of the main strategies used in neuroscientific psychiatry research, in tandem particularly with in vitro imaging and molecular genetics.

Acknowledgements
I am grateful to the Wellcome Trust, Medical Research Council and Stanley Foundation for research support. Sharon Eastwood kindly helped with the photographic illustrations.

References

(1) Higgins GA, Mah VH. In situ hybridization approaches to human neurological disease. In: Conn PM, ed. *Methods in neurosciences, volume 1: Gene probes*. San Diego: Academic Press, 1989: 183–96.

(2) Harrison PJ, Pearson RCA. In situ hybridization histochemistry and the study of gene expression in human brain. *Prog Neurobiol* 1990; 34: 271–312.

(3) Emson P. In situ hybridization as a methodological tool for the neuroscientist. *Trends Neurosci* 1993; 16: 9–16.

(4) Harrison PJ, Pearson CA. Principles and practice of in situ hybridization histochemistry in neuropsychiatric research. In: Roberts GW, Polak J, eds. *Molecular neuropathology*. Cambridge: Cambridge University Press; 1995; 38–60.

(5) Harrison PJ, Pearson RCA. Gene expression and mental disease. *Psychol Med* 1989; 19: 813–19.

(6) Hyman BT, Wenninger JJ, Tanzi RE. Nonisotopic in situ hybridization of amyloid beta protein precursor in Alzheimer's disease: expression in neurofibrillary tangle bearing neurons and in the microenvironment surrounding senile plaques. *Mol Brain Res* 1993; 18: 253–8.

(7) Kiyama H, Emson PC, Tohyama M. Recent progress in the use of the technique of non-radioactive in situ hybridization histochemistry: new tools for molecular neurobiology. *Neurosci Res* 1990; 9: 1–21.

(8) Polak JM, Van Noorden S. *An introduction to immunocytochemistry: current techniques and problems*. Royal Microscopical Society Handbooks, volume 11, revised edition. Oxford: Oxford Science Publications, Oxford University Press; 1987.

(9) Rogers WT, Schwaber JS, Lewis ME. Quantitation of cellular resolution in

situ hybridization histochemistry in brain by image analysis. *Neurosci Lett* 1987; 82: 315–20.

(10) Miller MA, Urban JH, Dorsa DM. Quantification of mRNA in discrete cell groups of brain by in situ hybridization histochemistry. In Conn PM, ed. *Methods in neurosciences, volume 1: Gene probes.* San Diego: Academic Press; 1989: 164–82.

(11) Masseroli M, Bollea A, Bendotti C, Forloni G. In situ hybridization histochemistry quantification: automatic count on single cell in digital image. *J Neurosci Methods* 1993; 47: 93–103.

(12) Hargrove JL. Microcomputer-assisted kinetic modelling of mammalian gene expression. *FASEB J* 1993; 7: 1163–70.

(13) Breitbart RE, Andreadis A, Nadel-Ginard B. Alternative splicing: a ubiquitous mechanism for the generation of multiple protein isoforms from single genes. *Ann Rev Biochem* 1987; 56: 467–95.

(14) Rio DC. Splicing of pre-mRNA: mechanism, regulation and role in development. *Curr Opin Genet Dev* 1993; 3: 574–84.

(15) Nakanishi S. Molecular diversity of glutamate receptors and implications for brain function. *Science* 1992; 258: 597–603.

(16) Sommer B, Keinanen K, Verdoorn TA et al. Flip and flop: a cell-specific functional switch in glutamate-operated channels of the CNS. *Science* 1990; 249: 1580–5.

(17) Pellegrini-Giampietro DE, Bennett MVL, Zukin RS. Differential expression of three glutamate receptor genes in developing rat brain: an in situ hybridization study. *Proc Natl Acad Sci USA* 1991; 88: 4157–61.

(18) Eastwood SL, Burnet PWJ, Beckwith J, Kerwin RW, Harrison PJ. AMPA glutamate receptors and their flip and flop in RNAs in human hippocampus. *Neuroreport* 1995; 5: 1325–8.

(19) Farooqui AA, Horrocks LA. Excitatory amino acid receptors, neural membrane phospholipid metabolism and neurological disorders. *Brain Res Rev* 1991; 16: 171–91.

(20) Harrison PJ, Eastwood SL, Kerwin RW. Gene expression in Down's syndrome, Parkinson's disease and schizophrenia. In: Harrison PJ, ed. *Regulation of gene expression and brain function, Volume 6, Basic and clinical aspects of neuroscience.* Berlin: Springer Verlag/Sandoz 1994: 57–64.

(21) Gerfen CR, McGinty JF, Young WS III. Dopamine differentially regulates dynorphin, substance P, and enkephalin expression in striatal neurons: in situ hybridization histochemical analysis. *J Neurosci* 1991; 11: 1016–31.

(22) Eastwood SL, Burnet PWJ McDonald B, Clinton J, Harrison PJ. Synaptophysin gene expression in human brain. A quantitative in situ hybridization and immunocytochemical study. *Neuroscience* 1994; 59: 871–82.

(23) Fukamauchi F, Saunders PA, Hough C, Chuang D-M. Agonist-induced downregulation and antagonist-induced upregulation of m2 and m3 muscarinic acetylcholine receptor mRNA and protein in cultured cerebellar granule cells. *Mol Pharmacol* 1993; 44: 940–9.

(24) Barton AJL, Harrison PJ, Najlerahim A, Heffernan J, McDonald B, Robinson JR et al. Increased tau messenger RNA in Alzheimer's disease hippocampus. *Am J Pathol* 1991; 137: 497–502.

(25) Goedert M, Potier MC, Spillantini MG. Molecular neuropathology of

Alzheimer's disease. In: Kerwin RW, ed. *Neurobiology and psychiatry, volume 1*. Cambridge: Cambridge University Press; 1991: 95–122.

(26) Golde TE, Estus S, Usiak M, Younkin LH, Younkin SG. Expression of β amyloid protein precursor mRNAs: recognition of a novel alternatively spliced form and quantitation in Alzheimer's disease using PCR. *Neuron* 1990; 4: 253–67.

(27) Price RH, Mayer B, Beitz AJ. Nitric oxide synthase neurons in rat brain express more NMDA receptor mRNA than non-NOS neurons. *NeuroReport* 1993; 4: 807–10.

(28) Normand E, Bloch B. Simultaneous detection of two messenger RNAs in the central nervous system: a simple two-step in situ hybridization procedure using a combination of radioactive and non-radioactive probes. *J Histochem Cytochem* 191; 39: 1575–8.

(29) Masliah E, Fagan AM, Terry RD et al. Reactive synaptogenesis assessed by synaptophysin immunoreactivity is associated with GAP-43 in the dentate gyrus of the adult rat. *Exp Neurol* 1991; 113: 131–42.

(30) Wahle P, Beckh S. A method of in situ hybridization combined with immunocytochemistry, histochemistry, and tract tracing to characterize the mRNA expressing cell types in heterogeneous neuronal populations. *J Neurosci Methods* 1992; 41: 153–66.

(31) Crick F, Jones EG. The backwardness of human neuroanatomy. *Nature* 1993; 361: 109–10.

(32) Rogers AW. *Techniques of autoradiography*, 3rd edition. Amsterdam: Elsevier; 1979.

(33) Markham A. The polymerase chain reaction. *Br Med J* 1993; 306: 441–6.

(34) Komminboth P, Long AA. In-situ polymerase chain reaction. An overview of methods, applications and limitations of a new molecular technique. *Virchows Arch B Cell Pathol* 1993; 64: 67–73.

(35) Kitazawa S, Kitazawa R, Yao C-H, Maeda S. In situ hybridization at electron microscopic level. *Acta Histochem Cytochem* 1993; 26: 295–301.

(36) Steward O, Banker GA. Getting the message from the gene to the synapse: sorting and intracellular transport of RNA in neurons. *Trends Neurosci* 1992; 15: 180–6.

(37) Kleiman R, Banker G, Steward O. Differential subcellular localization of particular mRNAs in hippocampal neurons in culture. *Neuron* 1990; 5: 821–30.

(38) Chicurel ME, Terrian DM, Potter H. mRNA at the synapse: analysis of a synaptosomal preparation enriched in hippocampal dendritic spines. *J Neurosci* 1993; 13: 14054–63.

(39) Mohr E, Richter D. Diversity of mRNAs in the axonal compartment of peptidergic neurons in the rat. *Eur J Neurosci* 1992; 4: 870–6.

(40) Surmeier DJ, Reiner A, Levine MS, Ariano MA. Are neostriatal dopamine receptors co-localized? *Trends Neurosci* 1993; 16: 299–305.

(41) Harrison PJ. On the neuropathology of schizophrenia and its dementia: neurodevelopmental, neurodegenerative, or both? *Neurodegeneration* 1995 (in press).

(42) Harrison PJ, Burnet PWJ. Antisense as an explanatory, experimental and therapeutic tool for psychiatric disorders. *Psychol Med* 1994; 24: 275–9.

(43) Wahlstedt C, Golanov E, Yamamoto S et al. Antisense oligodeoxynucleotides to NMDA-R1 receptor channel protect cortical neurons from excitotoxicity and reduce focal ischemic infarctions. *Nature* 1993; 363: 260–3.
(44) Somerville MJ, Percy ME, Bergeron C, Yoong LKK, Grima EA, McLachlan DRC. Localization and quantitation of 68 kDa neurofilament and superoxide dismutase-1 mRNA in Alzheimer brain. *Mol Brain Res* 1991; 9: 1–8.
(45) Jones EG, Hendry SHC, Liu X-L, Hodgins S, Potkin SG, Tourtellotte WW. A method for fixation of previously fresh-frozen human adult and fetal brains that preserves histological quality and immunoreactivity. *J Neurosci Methods* 1992; 44: 133–44.
(46) Harrison PJ, Procter AW, Barton AJL, Lowe SL, Najlerahim A, Bertolucci P et al. Terminal coma affects messenger RNA detection in post mortem human temporal cortex. *Mol Brain Res* 1991; 9: 161–4.
(47) Burke WJ, O'Malley K, Chung HD, Harmon SK, Miller P, Berg L. Effect of pre- and postmortem variables on specific mRNA levels in human brain. *Mol Brain Res* 1991; 11: 37–41.
(48) Barton AJL, Pearson RCA, Najlerahim A, Harrison PJ. Pre and post mortem influences on brain RNA. *J Neurochem* 1993; 61: 1–11.
(49) Leonard S, Logel J, Luthman D, Casanova M, Kirch D, Freedman R. Biological stability of mRNA isolated from human postmortem brain collections. *Biol Psychiat* 1993; 33: 456–66.
(50) Carpenter WT, Buchanan RW, Kirkpatrick B, Tamminga C, Wood F. Strong inference, theory testing, and the neuroanatomy of schizophrenia. *Arch Gen Psychiat* 1993; 50: 825–31.
(51) Kerwin RW. Glutamate receptors, microtubule associated proteins and developmental anomaly in schizophrenia: an hypothesis. *Psychol Med* 1993; 23: 547–51.
(52) Harrison PJ. Expression of the β amyloid precursor protein gene and the pathogenesis of Alzheimer's disease. In: Harrison PJ, ed. *Regulation of gene expression and brain function, Volume 6, Basic and clinical aspects of neuroscience.* Berlin: Springer/Verlag/Sandoz 1994: 48–56.
(53) Schmechel DE, Goldgaber D, Burkhart DS, Gilbert JR, Gadjusek DC, Roses AD. Cellular localization of messenger RNA encoding amyloid beta-protein in normal tissue and Alzheimer disease. *Alz Dis Assoc Disorders* 1988; 2: 96–111.
(54) Banati RB, Gehrmann J, Czech C et al. Early and rapid de novo synthesis of Alzheimer βA4-amyloid precursor protein (APP) in activated microglia. *Glia* 1993; 9: 199–210.
(55) Cohen ML, Golde TE, Usiak ME, Younkin LH, Younkin SG. In situ hybridization of nucleus basalis neurons shows increased beta-amyloid mRNA in Alzheimer's disease. *Proc Natl Acad Sci USA* 1988; 85: 1227–31.
(56) Palmert MR, Golde TE, Cohen ML et al. Amyloid protein precursor messenger RNAs: differential expression in Alzheimer's disease. *Science* 1988; 241: 1080–4.
(57) Harrison PJ, Procter AW, Bowen DM, Barton AJL, Pearson RCA. The effects of Alzheimer's disease, other dementias and premortem course upon amyloid β precursor protein messenger RNAs in frontal cortex. *J Neurochem* 1994; 62: 635–44.

(58) Roberts GW, Nash M, Ince PG, Royston MC, Gentleman SM. On the origin of Alzheimer's disease: a hypothesis. *NeuroReport* 1993; 4: 7–9.
(59) Johnson SA, McNeil T, Cordell B, Finch CE. Relation of neuronal APP751/APP695 mRNA ratio and neuritic plaque density in Alzheimer's disease. *Science* 1990; 248: 854–7.
(60) Oyama F, Shimada H, Oyama R, Titani K, Ihara Y. Differential expression of β amyloid protein precursor (APP) and tau mRNA in the aged human brain: individual variability and correlation between APP-751 and four-repeat tau. *J Neuropathol Exp Neurol* 1991; 50: 560–78.
(61) Hardy JA, Allsop D. Amyloid deposition as the central event in the aetiology of Alzheimer's disease. *Trends Pharmacol Sci* 1991; 12: 363–8.
(62) Selkoe DJ. Physiological production of the β-amyloid protein and the mechanism of Alzheimer's disease. *Trends Neurosci* 1993; 16: 403–9.
(63) Harrison PJ, Barton AJL , McDonald B, Pearson RCA. Alzheimer's disease: specific increases of a G protein subunit ($G_s\alpha$) mRNA in hippocampal and cortical neurons. *Mol Brain Res* 1991; 10: 71–81.
(64) Strada O, Vyas S, Hirsch EC et al. Decreased choline acetyltransferase mRNA expression in the nucleus basalis of Meynert in Alzheimer disease: an in situ hybridization study. *Proc Natl Acad Sci USA* 1992; 89: 9549–53.
(65) Kerwin RW, Patel S, Meldrum BS. Autoradiographic localisation of the glutamate receptor system in control and schizophrenic post-mortem hippocampal formation. *Neuroscience* 1990; 39: 25–32.
(66) Harrison PJ, McLaughlin D, Kerwin RW. Decreased hippocampal expression of a glutamate receptor gene in schizophrenia. *Lancet* 1991; 337: 450–2.
(67) Royston MC, Simpson MDC. Post mortem neurochemistry of schizophrenia. In Kerwin RW, ed. *Neurobiology and psychiatry, volume 1.* Cambridge: Cambridge University Press; 1991: 1–14.
(68) HIll WD, Arai M, Cohen JA, Trojanowski JQ. Neurofilament mRNA is reduced in Parkinson's disease substantia nigra pars compacta neurons. *J Comp Neurol* 1993; 329: 328–36.
(69) Kastner A, Hirsch EC, Agid Y, Javoy-Agid F. Tyrosine hydroxylase protein and messenger RNA in the dopaminergic nigral neurons of patients with Parkinson's disease. *Brain Res* 1993; 606: 341–5.
(70) Goate A, Chartier-Harlin MC, Mullan M, Brown J, Crawford F, Fidani L et al. Segregation of a missense mutation in the amyloid precursor protein gene with familial Alzheimer's disease. *Nature* 1991; 349: 704–6.
(71) Tanzi R, Hyman BT. Alzheimer mutation. *Nature* 1991; 350: 564.
(72) Harrison PJ, Barton AJL, Pearson RCA. Expression of amyloid beta-protein mRNAs in familial Alzheimer's disease. *NeuroReport* 1990; 2: 152–5.
(73) Scott J. Apolipoprotein E and Alzheimer's disease. *Lancet* 1993; 342: 696.
(74) Wisniewski T, Frangione B. Apolipoprotein E: a pathological chaperone in patients with cerebral and systemic amyloid. *Neurosci Lett* 1991; 135: 235–8.
(75) Namba Y, Tomonaga M, Kawasaki H, Otomo E, Ikeda K. Apolipoprotein E immunoreactivity in cerebral deposits and neurofibrillary tangles in Alzheimer's disease and kuru plaque amyloid in Creutzfeldt–Jakob disease. *Brain Res* 1991; 541: 163–6.

(76) Diedrich JF, Minnigan H, Carp RI, Whittaker JN, Race R, Frey W II, Haase AT. Neuropathological changes in scrapie and Alzheimer's disease are associated with increased expression of apolipoprotein E and cathepsin D in astrocytes. *J Virol* 1991; 65: 4759–68.
(77) Huntington's Disease Collaborative Group. A novel gene containing a trinucleotide repeat that is expanded and unstable on Huntington's disease chromosomes. *Cell* 1993; 72: 971–83.
(78) Li SH, Schilling G, Young WS III, Li XJ, Margolis RL, Stine OC et al. Huntington's disease gene (IT15) is widely expressed in human and rat tissues. *Neuron* 1993; 11: 985–93.
(79) Strong TV, Tagle DA, Valdes JM, Elmer LW, Boehm K, Swaroop M et al. Widespread expression of the human and rat Huntington's disease gene in brain and nonneural tissues. *Nature Genet* 1993; 5: 259–65.
(80) Richardson EP Jr. Huntington's disease: some recent neuropathological studies. *Neuropath Appl Neurobiol* 1990; 16: 451–60.
(81) Collinge J, Curtis D. The current literature: decreased hippocampal expression of a glutamate receptor gene in schizophrenia. *Br J Psychiat* 1991; 159: 857–9.
(82) Mulcrone J, Whatley S. The application of differential cloning techniques in post mortem studies of neuropsychiatric disorders: a way ahead. *Psychol Med* 1993; 23: 825–9.
(83) LeBlanc AC, Poduslo JF. Regulation of apolipoprotein E gene expression after injury of the rat sciatic nerve. *J Neurosci Res* 190; 25: 162–70.
(84) Poirier J, Hess M, May PC, Finch CE. Astrocytic apolipoprotein E mRNA and GFAP mRNA in hippocapus after entorhinal cortex lesioning. *Mol Brain Res* 1991; 11: 97–106.
(85) Scott JN, Parhad IM, Clark AW. β Amyloid precursor protein gene is differentially expressed in axotomised sensory and motor systems. *Mol Brain Res* 1991; 10: 315–25.
(86) Wallace WC, Bragin V, Robakis NK et al. Increased biosynthesis of Alzheimer amyloid precursor protein in the cerebral cortex of rats with lesions of the nucleus basalis of Meynert. *Mol Brain Res* 1991; 10: 173–8.
(87) Sola C, Garcia-Ladona FJ, Sarasa M, Mengod G, Probst A. βAPP gene expression is increased in the rat brain after motor neuron axotomy. *Eur J Neurosci* 1993; 5: 795–808.
(88) Bernard V, Le Moine C, Bloch B. Striatal neurons express increased level of dopamine D2 receptor mRNA in response to haloperidol treatment: a quantitative in situ hybridization study. *Neuroscience* 1991; 45: 117–26.
(89) Harrison PJ. Effects of neuroleptics on neuronal and synaptic structure. In: Barnes TRE, ed. *Antipsychotic drugs and their side-effects*. London: Academic Press; 1993: 100–9.
(90) Eastwood SL, Story P, Burnet PWJ, Heath P, Harrison PJ. Differential changes in glutamate receptor subunit messenger RNAs in rat brain after haloperidol treatment. *J Psychopharmacol* 1994; 8: 196–203.
(91) Masliah E, Terry RD. The role of synaptic proteins in the pathogenesis of disorders of the central nervous system. *Brain Pathol* 1993; 3: 77–85.

Index

Index